Video Atlas of Acute Ischemic Stroke Intervention

Maxim Mokin, MD, PhD, FSVIN
Associate Professor
Department of Neurosurgery and Brain Repair
Director of Neuroendovascular Fellowship Program
University of South Florida
Tampa, Florida, USA

Elad I. Levy, MD, MBA, FACS, FAHA
Professor and Chair
Department of Neurosurgery and Radiology
State University of New York
SUNY Distinguished Professor
Director, American Board of Neurological Surgery
Director of Stroke Services
Kaleida Health
Buffalo, New York, USA

Adnan H. Siddiqui, MD, PhD, FACS, FAHA, FAANS
Professor and Vice Chair
Department of Neurosurgery and Radiology
Director of Neuroendovascular Fellowship Program
State University of New York
Buffalo, New York, USA

311 illustrations

Thieme
New York • Stuttgart • Delhi • Rio de Janeiro

Library of Congress Cataloging-in-Publication Data is available with the publisher.

Important note: Medicine is an ever-changing science undergoing continual development. Research and clinical experience are continually expanding our knowledge, in particular our knowledge of proper treatment and drug therapy. Insofar as this book mentions any dosage or application, readers may rest assured that the authors, editors, and publishers have made every effort to ensure that such references are in accordance with **the state of knowledge at the time of production of the book**.

Nevertheless, this does not involve, imply, or express any guarantee or responsibility on the part of the publishers in respect to any dosage instructions and forms of applications stated in the book. **Every user is requested to examine carefully** the manufacturers' leaflets accompanying each drug and to check, if necessary, in consultation with a physician or specialist, whether the dosage schedules mentioned therein or the contraindications stated by the manufacturers differ from the statements made in the present book. Such examination is particularly important with drugs that are either rarely used or have been newly released on the market. Every dosage schedule or every form of application used is entirely at the user's own risk and responsibility. The authors and publishers request every user to report to the publishers any discrepancies or inaccuracies noticed. If errors in this work are found after publication, errata will be posted at www.thieme.com on the product description page.

Some of the product names, patents, and registered designs referred to in this book are in fact registered trademarks or proprietary names even though specific reference to this fact is not always made in the text. Therefore, the appearance of a name without designation as proprietary is not to be construed as a representation by the publisher that it is in the public domain.

Thieme addresses people of all gender identities equally. We encourage our authors to use gender-neutral or gender-equal expressions wherever the context allows.

Thieme Publishers New York
333 Seventh Avenue, 18th Floor
New York, NY 10001, USA
www.thieme.com
+1 800 782 3488, customerservice@thieme.com

Illustrations: Jennifer Pryll
Cover design: © Thieme
Cover image source: © Thieme/Jennifer Pryll
Typesetting by TNQ Technologies, India

Printed in USA by King Printing Company, Inc.   5 4 3 2 1

ISBN: 978-1-68420-249-2

Also available as an e-book:
eISBN (PDF): 978-1-68420-250-8
eISBN (epub): 978-1-63853-705-2

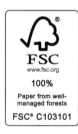

FSC
www.fsc.org
100%
Paper from well-managed forests
FSC® C103101

I dedicate this work to my mentors from Buffalo. An unexpected stroke neurology rotation at the former Millard Fillmore Gates Circle Hospital as an intern led to the most amazing clinical and research experience—an experience that forever shaped my future.

Maxim Mokin

This book is dedicated to the unyielding support, generosity, and love from my caring and benevolent wife, Cindy, and three children, Bennett, Hannon, and Lauren. To my parents, who taught me by example that passion, grit, and sacrifice are the key components to everything worth accomplishing. And to all the patients who have taught me so much through their courage.

Elad I. Levy

I dedicate this work to patients who have suffered stroke. Their struggle and strife provide the fuel that has powered this work. Their fortitude and resolve inspire all of us in the field of stroke care. To all the women and men who have endured.

Adnan H. Siddiqui

Contents

Contents

Videos

Foreword

Endovascular treatment of acute ischemic stroke is a rapidly evolving field. Propelled by the multitude of randomized trials attesting to the highly effective nature of this treatment, disruptive technological advances have led not only to an ever-increasing complexity of endovascular reperfusion therapies but also to an expansion of the treatment-eligible patient population. The staggering amount of emerging new information required for the neurointerventional practitioner to stay up to date with these rapidly evolving developments necessitates educational material that can be updated on an ongoing basis and that incorporates hands-on information regarding technical aspects of interventional stroke procedures (including technical pitfalls and complications) along with an overview of the most useful tools of the trade in conjunction with information regarding pre- and postprocedural care. Educational material compiled by the group of leaders in the field of acute stroke interventions has the potential to be one of the most effective tools for continuing education that the neuro-interventional practitioner and associated staff have at their disposal. It is these leaders who comprise the authorship of the *Video Atlas of Acute Ischemic Stroke Intervention*.

This carefully selected collection of routinely encountered cases delivered primarily in video format, accompanied by expert comments and clinical vignettes, is a much-needed and timely contribution that fills a real void in education and knowledge as it represents a "living" and comprehensive overview of technical aspects related to acute stroke interventions. Given the complexity of acute stroke care and the fact that the knowledge included in this atlas can be life (or brain) saving, every practitioner involved in the interventional care of patients with acute stroke could benefit from having a copy of the *Video Atlas of Acute Ischemic Stroke Intervention* readily available.

Tudor G. Jovin, MD
Chair, Department of Neurology
Cooper University Hospital
Professor of Neurology
Cooper Medical School of Rowan University
Director
Cooper Neurological Institute
New Jersey, USA

Preface

Since the publication of the *Video Atlas of Neuroendovascular Procedures,* we have received a number of comments from the readers asking for more in-depth coverage of certain topics. Of those, endovascular treatment of acute ischemic stroke received the most attention. This is not surprising, considering a recent revolution in the effective management of this devastating brain pathology with the use of modern technological advances. Therefore, in this *Video Atlas of Acute Ischemic Stroke Intervention,* we concentrated our current knowledge and decades of experience in acute stroke treatment and device innovations in Buffalo to help the readers at various levels of training become familiar with the wide repertoire of techniques available in the neurointerventional suite.

Following the traditional format of a video atlas describing clinical and neuroimaging findings, procedure planning, complications avoidance, and management, which proved to be highly successful among our readers, we continue to focus on individually narrated high-definition videos of angiographic and procedural cases describing step-by-step components of the procedure. In this atlas, we provide comprehensive coverage of the most common approaches to the endovascular treatment of acute stroke consisting of aspiration and stent-retriever thrombectomy of proximal, distal, and tandem occlusions. We also provide an overview of tips and tricks to the most challenging and less common pathologies, including arterial dissection, atherosclerosis, and venous strokes, as well as review in detail the importance of arterial access, unmet need in current devices, and ways to overcome such challenges. Several cases are dedicated to the recognition and management of complications that might be encountered during these emergent procedures.

We hope that you find this new book a helpful go-to resource for a variety of clinical scenarios that can often unexpectedly arise when managing acute stroke cases.

Maxim Mokin, MD, PhD, FSVIN
Elad I. Levy, MD, MBA, FACS, FAHA
Adnan H. Siddiqui, MD, PhD, FACS, FAHA, FAANS

Acknowledgments

We thank medical illustrator Jennifer Pryll for continuous work and collaboration with us for preparing the high-quality illustrations that are so helpful in explaining and emphasizing the key aspects of complex neurointerventional procedures. We also thank medical illustrator Paul H. Dressel, BFA, for preparing the technical videos and procedural images that are key components of this interactive video atlas and Debi Zimmer for providing the necessary editorial assistance to ensure accuracy and consistency of every book chapter. We are very grateful for the ongoing support from the Thieme team, beginning from the early concept development of this video atlas series, intricate editorial process, to final publication. We greatly appreciate tremendous support from the nurses and technicians at Gates Vascular Institute, Kaleida Health. We are forever thankful to the many current and former residents and neuroendovascular fellows from our program who we proudly refer to as the Buffalo family. Lastly, we are deeply indebted to Dr. Nick Hopkins for his vision, perseverance, and uncanny ability to stimulate multidisciplinary collaborations. This work would not have been possible without Nick's continuous support and leadership.

Maxim Mokin, MD, PhD, FSVIN
Elad I. Levy, MD, MBA, FACS, FAHA
Adnan H. Siddiqui, MD, PhD, FACS, FAHA, FAANS

Contributors

Jason M. Davies, MD, PhD
Assistant Professor
Departments of Neurosurgery and Biomedical Informatics
State University of New York;
Director of Cerebrovascular Microsurgery;
Director of Endoscopy, Kalcida Health
Buffalo, New York, USA

Kenneth V. Snyder, MD, PhD
Associate Professor
Department of Neurosurgery and Radiology
State University of New York;
Vice-President of Physician Quality for Kaleida Health
Buffalo, New York, USA

Muhammad Waqas, MBBS
Neuroendovascular Fellow
Department of Neurosurgery
State University of New York
Buffalo, New York, USA

1 Clinical and Imaging Evaluation

General Description

An abundance of medical information has been written about the various clinical and imaging methodologies for the evaluation of a patient for endovascular thrombectomy (ET). This chapter represents a more pragmatic approach to the evaluation of acute ischemic stroke (AIS) in a patient with a suspected large vessel occlusion (LVO). Here, we discuss how to recognize and confirm the presence of LVO based on the clinical presentation and review the minimal imaging criteria necessary to decide whether to bring the patient to the angiography suite for ET.

Keywords: ASPECTS, large vessel occlusion, NIHSS, perfusion

1.1 Clinical Evaluation

- Prehospital stroke screening tools essentially serve two tasks: (1) to distinguish stroke from stroke-like mimics (such as encephalopathy or hypoglycemia) and (2) to identify stroke patients with a high probability of having an LVO. These tools are most relevant in the prehospital setting when emergency medical personnel determine the most appropriate type of stroke center for the triage of a patient with a suspected stroke.
- The Face Arm Speech Test (FAST) and Cincinnati Prehospital Stroke Scale (CPSS) are examples of stroke screen tools that incorporate facial palsy, motor arm, and dysarthria. The Los Angeles Motor Scale (LAMS) and the Rapid Arterial oCclusion Evaluation (RACE) are examples of LVO detection scales.
- The National Institute of Health Stroke Scale (NIHSS) is the AIS severity score that is most relevant to the in-hospital setting (▶ Table 1.1). This is a uniform language that allows medical providers to accurately gauge stroke severity, communicate with each other, and make treatment decisions. Diligent documentation of baseline NIHSS score allows timely recognition of early neurological deterioration, alerting the neurointerventionist of possible complications such as reperfusion hemorrhage or reocclusion.
- Most patients with AIS from LVO eligible for ET will have an NIHSS score within the 10 to 25 range. Patients with "mild" symptoms defined as NIHSS score < 6 may harbor an LVO or a more distal medium vessel occlusion (MeVO); the decision to proceed with ET in such patients requires a more thorough consideration of the associated risks and benefits.

Table 1.1 The National Institutes of Health Stroke Scale (NIHSS)

Category	Score description
Level of consciousness (LOC)	0—alert 1—easily arousable by minor stimulation 2—not alert, requires repeated stimulation 3—unresponsive/flaccid
LOC Questions	0—answers both questions correctly 1—one question correctly 2—answers neither question correctly
LOC One-step commands	0—performs both tasks correctly 1—performs one command correctly 2—performs neither command correctly
Gaze	0—normal gaze 1—partial gaze palsy 2—forced deviation or total palsy
Vision	0—no visual loss 1—partial hemianopia 2—complete hemianopia 3—bilateral hemianopia or cortical blindness
Face	0—normal 1—minor paralysis 2—partial paralysis (lower face) 3—complete paralysis (of one or both side)
Motor arm	0—no drift 1—drift 2—some effort against gravity 3—no effort against gravity 4—no movement
Motor leg	0—no drift 1—drift 2—some effort against gravity 3—no effort against gravity 4—no movement
Limb ataxia	0—absent 1—present in one limb 2—present in two limbs
Sensory	0—normal 1—mild or moderate sensory loss 2—severe or total sensory loss
Language	0—normal 1—mild or moderate aphasia 2—severe aphasia 3—global aphasia or patient is mute
Dysarthria	0—normal 1—mild or moderate dysarthria 2—severe dysarthria
Extinction and inattention	0—normal 1—deficit in one modality 2—deficit in more than one modality or profound deficit

Source: Adapted from https://stroke.nih.gov/resources/scale.htm

1.2 Imaging Evaluation

- Brain noncontrast computed tomography (NCCT) scan allows rapid differentiation between AIS and brain hemorrhage. This simple imaging modality is an ideal choice in many emergency departments (ED).
- Just like the NIHSS score allows team members to accurately communicate the degree of clinical stroke severity, the Alberta Stroke Program Early CT Score (ASPECTS) is a common imaging scoring system to describe the extent of early stroke on CT (▶ Fig. 1.1).
- In many cases, NCCT combined with computed tomography angiography (CTA) to detect the location and extent of LVO will provide the minimum information needed to determine if ET is indicated (▶ Fig. 1.2).
- Additional imaging modalities, such as brain perfusion (mainly in the form of computed tomography perfusion [CTP]) or magnetic resonance imaging (MRI), are often not necessary (▶ Fig. 1.2 and ▶ Fig. 1.3). ET is capable of greatly reducing disability and mortality in a wide range of patients including those with various degrees of baseline stroke burden and LVO location, all of which can be reliably assessed with CT and CTA alone. Of course, unique clinical scenarios exist when additional imaging is needed (▶ Fig. 1.4).

1.3 Pearls and Pitfalls

- ASPECTS calculated on CT with customized window width/level setting adjustments will improve the sensitivity for detection of early ischemic changes (▶ Fig. 1.1).
- In addition to estimating the extent of stroke burden, NCCT may identify a hyperdense vessel sign suggestive of LVO (▶ Fig. 1.5) or alert to an underlying calcified plaque and guide the operator in choosing the most appropriate intervention.
- In addition to confirming or excluding LVO, CTA provides information about variations in aortic arch anatomy and tortuosity and stenosis or occlusion of extracranial vessels. CTA also helps evaluate the status of the circle of Willis and recognize anatomical intracranial variants. These critical points may dictate the choice of arterial access (femoral vs. radial), guide catheter, and thrombectomy device and are discussed further in Chapter 2 "Arterial Access" and Chapter 3 "Challenging Access."
- The accuracy of CTA and CTP imaging depends on the quality and timing of contrast injection and image acquisition. This is especially important for accurate interpretation of CTP (▶ Fig. 1.6). CTP imaging has been mainly validated for acute anterior circulation LVO. Its clinical relevance for cases of chronic occlusion, significant stenosis, or posterior circulation strokes needs to be considered with caution (▶ Fig. 1.7).

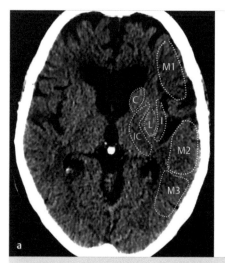
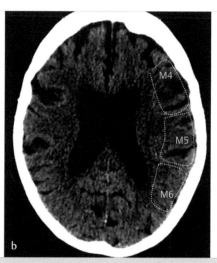
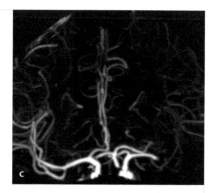
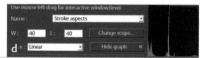

Fig. 1.1 Alberta Stroke Program Early CT Score (ASPECTS). Noncontrast computed tomography (NCCT), axial view. **(a)** Ganglionic and **(b)** supraganglionic levels. The scan is assigned a score ranging from 0 to 10 using 10 standard regions representing distinct middle cerebral artery (MCA) territories. A cumulative score is calculated based on the evidence (score of 0) or lack of (score of 1) early ischemic changes in each territory. C, caudate; IC, internal capsule; L, lentiform nucleus; I, insula; M1–3, ganglionic cortical regions; M4–6, supraganglionic cortical regions. Regions M4 and M5 contain early ischemic changes; thus, the total ASPECTS is 8. **(c)** Computed tomography angiography (CTA), three-dimensional (3D) reconstruction, demonstrating a left M1 occlusion. **(d)** Screen shot example of windowing and leveling used in this case. Here, Window 40/Level 40 is selected for the best visualization of early ischemic changes. Optimal stroke windows will depend on visual preferences and thus may be different. W: 35–40/L: 35–40 are commonly used.

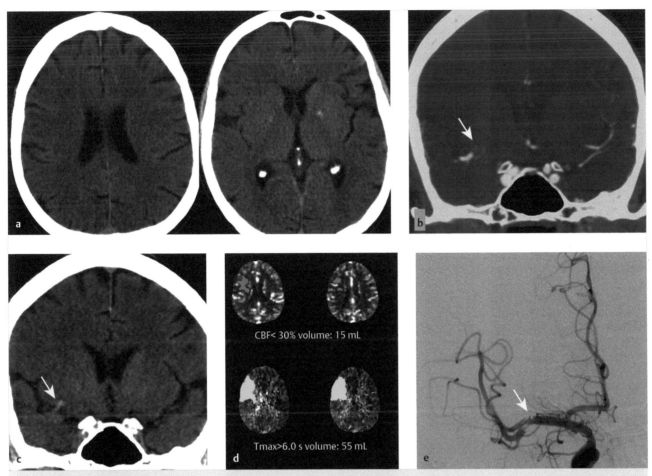

Fig. 1.2 Noncontrast computed tomography (NCCT) and computed tomography angiography (CTA) for detecting middle carotid artery (MCA) occlusion. **(a)** NCCT, axial view (left image—supraganglionic level, right image—ganglionic level). Minimal early ischemic changes are present. Alberta Stroke Program Early CT Score (ASPECTS) is above 6. **(b)** CTA, coronal view, showing a filling defect at the right M1 bifurcation representing a fresh clot (*arrow*). This patient has an National Institutes of Health Stroke Scale (NIHSS) score of 16 (neglect, right gaze preference, and left hemiparesis). The imaging data obtained in **(a)** and **(b)** are sufficient to determine the eligibility of this patient for endovascular thrombectomy (ET). **(c)** NCCT, coronal view, showing a hyperdense MCA sign (*arrow*). With such a high NIHSS score, the decision to proceed with ET is even reasonable without obtaining CTA, which becomes relevant for cases in which CTA is not readily available. **(d)** Computed tomography perfusion (CTP), automated processing with RapidAI software (iSchemaView), depicting an M2 MCA territory region with abnormal perfusion (*green*—ischemic penumbra, *magenta*—ischemic core). Although this imaging pattern proves that the patient is eligible for ET, the same clinical decision to treat with ET can be reached without CTP. A more harmful clinical scenario would be to obtain CTP showing an "unfavorable" imaging profile and use this information to exclude the patient from ET all together. **(e)** Digital subtraction angiography (DSA), right internal carotid artery (ICA) injection, anteroposterior (AP) view, confirming a "saddle" embolus in the MCA bifurcation extending into both M2 branches (*arrow*).

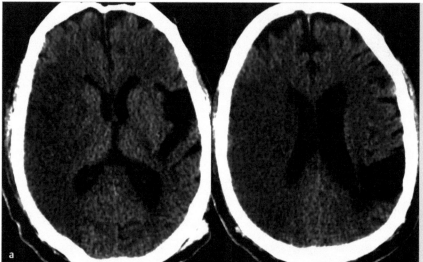

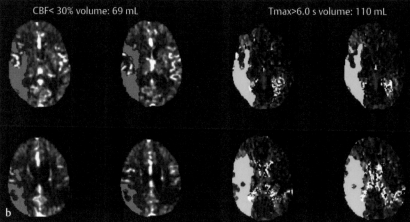

CBF< 30% volume: 69 mL — Tmax>6.0 s volume: 110 mL

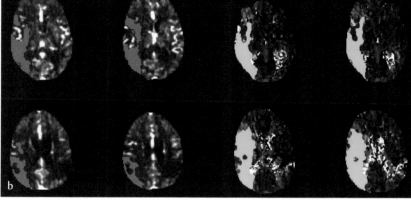

Fig. 1.3 Example of M1 occlusion with poor Alberta Stroke Program Early CT Score (ASPECTS). **(a)** Noncontrast computed tomography (NCCT), axial view (left image—ganglionic level, right image—supraganglionic level). In this case of wake-up right internal carotid artery (ICA) occlusion, extensive ischemic changes of the entire middle carotid artery (MCA) territory are present. The ASPECTS is 1 (the caudate region is the only one without signs of ischemia). Endovascular thrombectomy (ET) in this case is futile. **(b)** Computed tomography perfusion (CTP), showing a large MCA territory region with abnormal perfusion (*green*—ischemic penumbra, *magenta*—ischemic core). In this case, the extent of the perfusion imaging core is underestimated as ischemic damage of M4–6 MCA regions is clearly seen on NCCT already.

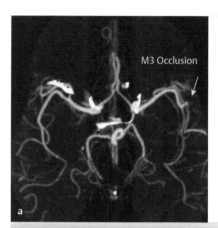

M3 Occlusion

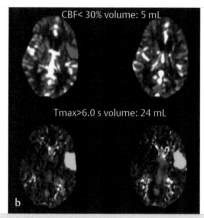

CBF< 30% volume: 5 mL

Tmax>6.0 s volume: 24 mL

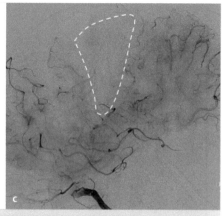

Fig. 1.4 Example of distal middle cerebral artery (MCA) occlusion recognized with computed tomography perfusion (CTP). **(a)** Computed tomography angiography (CTA), three-dimensional (3D) reconstruction. Left MCA M3 occlusion (*arrow*) was initially missed upon initial CTA review and not detected by automated software analysis (RapidAI [iSchemaView]) for large vessel occlusion (LVO) detection. **(b)** CTP, showing a small distal MCA territory region with abnormal perfusion corresponding to the motor cortex (*green*—ischemic penumbra, *magenta*—ischemic core). The patient's symptoms of contralateral weakness and the CTP finding prompted a more careful review of the CTA study, and this time a possible left M3 occlusion was recognized. **(c)** Digital subtraction angiography (DSA), lateral view, left internal carotid artery (ICA) injection, capillary phase, demonstrating a wedge-shaped perfusion deficit (*dashed region*) corresponding to an M3-branch occlusion. This was subsequently treated with local intra-arterial (IA) tissue plasminogen activator (tPA) infusion (not shown).

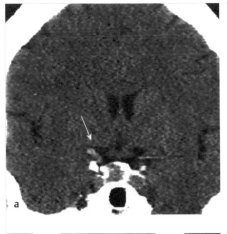

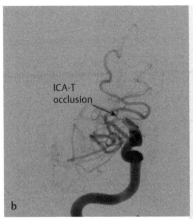

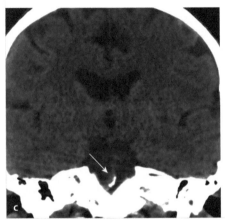

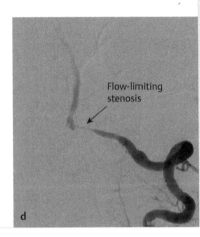

Fig. 1.5 Examples of noncontrast computed tomography (NCCT) alone demonstrating large vessel occlusion (LVO). **(a)** NCCT, coronal view, showing a hyperdense vessel sign (*arrow*). This represents an acute clot in the Internal carotid artery (ICA) terminus. There was a delay in establishing intravenous access for the computed tomography angiography (CTA) study. The patient was immediately taken to the angiography suite where an endovascular thrombectomy (ET) for an ICA terminus occlusion was performed. **(b)** Digital subtraction angiography (DSA), anteroposterior (AP) view, confirming right ICA terminus occlusion (*arrow*). **(c)** NCCT, coronal view, showing extensive calcifications of the proximal basilar artery (*arrow*) in a patient with posterior circulation stroke. **(d)** DSA, AP view, left vertebral artery (VA) injection, confirming critical left flow-limiting vertebrobasilar stenosis (*arrow*). Recognizing atherosclerosis as the underlying etiology of this lesion, acute stenting was chosen for treatment.

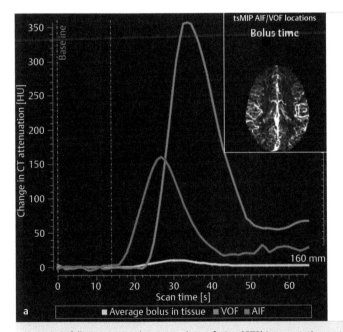

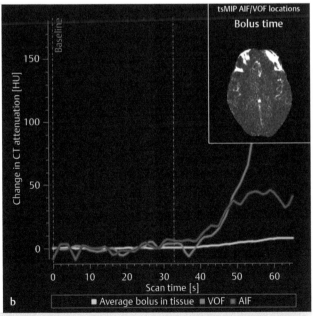

Fig. 1.6 Pitfalls in computed tomography perfusion (CTP) interpretation—arterial and venous curves. **(a)** Screenshot, automated arterial input function (AIF, *red curve*) and venous input function (VOF, *blue curve*). This is an example of good AIF and VOF placement and curves. The inset demonstrates arterial and venous placement of AIF and VOF, respectively. **(b)** Screenshot, showing nondiagnostic AIF (*red curve*) and VOF (*blue curve*). This can be a result of inappropriate placement of either AIF or VOF (which can be corrected by manual adjustment of placement), from poor timing of contrast injection, or simply poor contrast bolus.

2 Arterial Access

General Description

Arterial access is the first and often a key critical step in ensuring the successful outcome of a neuroendovascular procedure. Femoral artery (FA) access represents the most common choice among interventionists. However, radial artery (RA) access has become increasingly used for posterior circulation cases, as well as some anterior circulation strokes, such as those with challenging aortic arch anatomy. The ideal access approach should allow the operator to use the guide catheter of choice depending on the location of the large vessel occlusion (LVO), require minimal time to access the target vessel, and have low risk for access-site complications.

Keywords: Brachial artery, femoral artery, radial artery, ultrasound, vasospasm

2.1 Anatomical and Imaging Aspects

- When selecting the optimal arterial route for a particular stroke case, several factors should be taken into consideration, including the following:
  - Anterior versus posterior circulation. In general, RA is preferable for posterior circulation strokes. Left RA is preferred if the left vertebral artery (VA) is the dominant one.
  - In arterial circulation strokes, especially if balloon-guide catheter (BGC) use is planned, FA access with a 9-French (F) sheath may be preferable, although some operators have adapted to using RA access even if a BGC is used.
  - Aortic arch anatomy is critical in identifying cases where RA may be more beneficial, such as the presence of a bovine arch or the need to access the right carotid artery in a

patient with a type II or III arch (▶ Fig. 2.1). However, modern, highly trackable guide catheters (such as an 0.088-inch TracStar [Imperative Care] or AXS Infinity [Stryker]) help with fast, reliable transfemoral access even in such anatomically challenging cases. These unique situations are discussed in Chapter 3 "Challenging Access."

2.2 Technique and Key Steps—FA Access

- The optimal location of FA cannulation is below the origin of the inferior epigastric artery and above the FA bifurcation (▶ Fig. 2.2). Relying on palpation of the bony structures such as the anterior superior iliac spines to estimate the location of the inguinal ligament can be inaccurate. We prefer to visualize the femoral head with fluoroscopy using a hemostat, which helps us more accurately estimate the level of the needle puncture, followed by repeat fluoroscopy (▶ Fig. 2.2, ▶ Fig. 2.3). If the level of the puncture is suboptimal, this is an ideal opportunity to remove the micropuncture needle before exchanging it for a larger size dilator or placing a sheath.
- "High" access into the FA increases the risk of a retroperitoneal hematoma at that location, which can be life-threatening. "Low" access, below the FA bifurcation, can predispose to pseudoaneurysm formation, as well as interfere with safe use of closure devices.
- Because of the time-sensitive nature of the thrombectomy procedure, some operators perform femoral angiography at the end of the case. A low threshold for angiographic assessment of the FA should exist; if any resistance is encountered while accessing the FA or any concern for FA injury is present, angiography of the puncture site is needed.

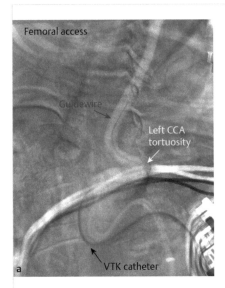
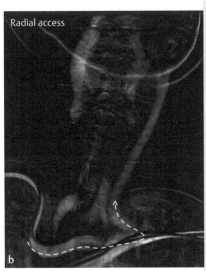

Fig. 2.1 An example of failed carotid artery access via a transfemoral route. **(a)** Roadmap, anteroposterior (AP) view, left common carotid artery injection. In this case, the transfemoral route is very challenging because of the combination of a type III arch and tortuosity of the proximal left common carotid artery (*yellow arrow*). Despite having the VTK catheter (*black arrow*; Cook Medical) in the left common carotid artery origin, any attempts to advance a 0.035-inch guidewire (*green arrow*; GlideWire [Terumo]) result in wire herniation. **(b)** Roadmap, AP view, left common carotid artery injection. Using a transradial approach, access to the left common carotid artery is less tortuous and thus more straightforward (indicated by the *yellow dashed line*). This is a common scenario in which recognizing such a challenging arch configuration before the case should prompt the interventionist to consider the RA as the first-line access approach.

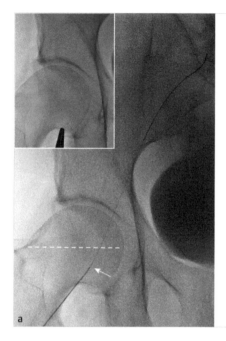
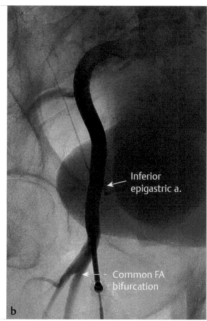

Fig. 2.2 Optimal level of femoral artery (FA) puncture. **(a)** Fluoroscopy, showing the level of the micropuncture needle accessing the FA (*arrow*). The *dashed line* is splitting the femoral head in half. Optimal localization of the puncture is at or just below the equator line of the femoral head. The inset shows the use of a hemostat to localize the femoral head. **(b)** Unsubstracted angiography, right common FA injection. The sheath is placed below the origin of the inferior epigastric artery (*solid arrow*) and above the common FA bifurcation (*dashed arrow*).

Inferior epigastric a.

Common FA bifurcation

2.3 Technique and Key Steps—RA Access

- The RA averages 2.6 mm in diameter. The use of ultrasound (U/S) (▶ Fig. 2.4) greatly increases the chance of successful puncture of the artery on the first attempt and reduces vasospasm and need for crossover to FA catheterization. A small size of the RA from a congenital anomaly, previous injury, or peripheral vascular disease should prompt evaluation of the ulnar artery and consideration of alternative access using that approach.
- The success rate of RA access can be increased by consistent preprocedure room setup, patient positioning, and use of U/S. The technique for RA access is described in ▶ Fig. 2.5 and ▶ Fig. 2.6. We commonly use 6F or 7F slender hydrophilic sheaths (Terumo) that do not require a dilator. An RA cocktail (2.5 mg of verapamil, 200 µg of nitroglycerin, and 3000 units of heparin) is administered through the RA sheath after its placement.
- If a long guide sheath is planned for access, it can be exchanged over the RA sheath. A variety of hydrophilic 6F inner diameter sheaths can be used, such as AXS Infinity (Stryker), Pinnacle Destination (Terumo), or Ashahi Fubuki (Ashahi Intecc), depending on the target location for the guide catheter.

2.4 Technique and Key Steps—Alternative Access

- Brachial artery access can be considered when the RA or ulnar artery cannot be safely catheterized, yet direct access to the subclavian artery is desired. Bedside U/S and radiographic guidance are needed for this access (▶ Fig. 2.7). The brachial artery, similar to its more distal branches, can be prone to vasospasm.
- Direct access to the internal carotid artery is usually performed as a last resort when all other attempts to obtain access have failed.

2.5 Pearls and Pitfalls

- Depending on the angiographic appearance of the FA, the use of a closure device may not be safe (▶ Fig. 2.8). Manual pressure at the access site can be less effective in a patient who was given a loading dose of glycoprotein IIb/IIIa inhibitors during the procedure or just completed a course of intravenous (IV) tissue plasminogen activator (tPA); in such cases, securing the sheath and removing it several hours later may be required.
- FA access can result in a life-threatening, albeit rare, complication. Groin hematoma can cause significant

blood loss (▶ Fig. 2.9). Major pain, an expanding palpable mass at the access site, or hemodynamic instability warrants immediate attention. Examination alone can often result in a diagnosis of groin hematoma; in some cases, computed tomography (CT) of the abdomen and pelvis or groin U/S is required to confirm the diagnosis.

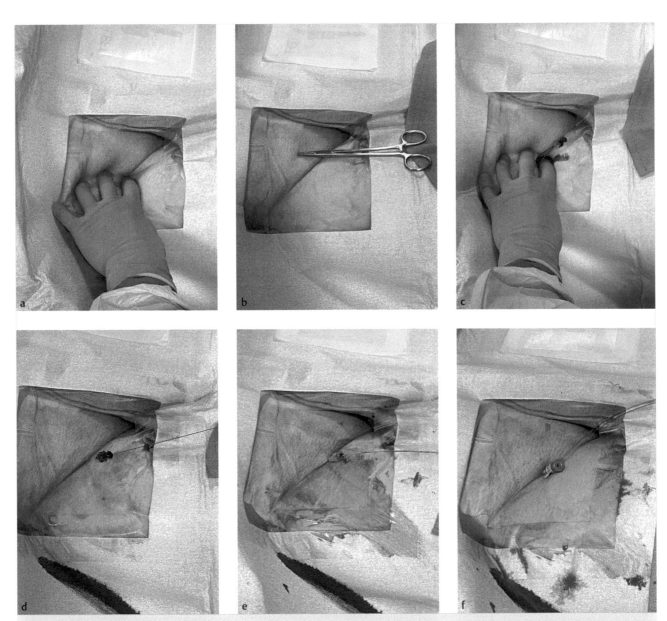

Fig. 2.3 Femoral artery (FA) access and sheath placement. **(a)** Palpation of the FA to evaluate pulse strength. **(b)** A hemostat is placed, and fluoroscopy is performed to localize the femoral head. **(c)** A 21-gauge (G) micropuncture needle (Cook Medical) is advanced at a 45-degree angle until blood return is seen. **(d)** An 0.018-inch, 40-cm guidewire (Cook Medical) is advanced, and its placement within the external iliac artery and away from side branches is confirmed with fluoroscopy (not shown). **(e)** The micropuncture needle is exchanged for a 5F dilator (Cook Medical). **(f)** Using a 0.035-inch J wire, an 8F short sheath (Terumo) is placed and connected to a saline flush. An 8F sheath will accommodate most 0.088-inch guide catheters that are routinely used for access during stroke interventions.

In most cases, successful hemostasis can be achieved by applying additional manual pressure. Reversal of anticoagulation and antiplatelets and a vascular surgery consultation may be required in some cases.

• Retroperitoneal hematomas can be more difficult to recognize with physical examination alone. They often result from "high stick" FA access (▶ Fig. 2.10) and warrant immediate abdomen and pelvis CT examination. Back pain is a red flag for this type of a hematoma. Unfortunately, many stroke patients may not be able to communicate their symptoms clearly, making careful angiographic assessment of FA access even more important.

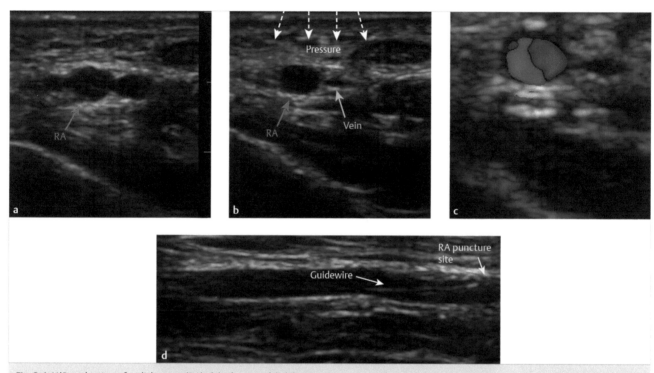

Fig. 2.4 U/S evaluation of radial artery (RA). **(a)** Ultrasound (U/S), transverse image, showing the typical appearance of the RA (*arrow*) and its associated vein. The scale bar on the right side is set at 10 mm. The RA size is adequate for access. **(b)** U/S, transverse image. The use of compression (indicated by the *white dashed arrows*) by the U/S probe will help to differentiate the RA (*red arrow*; will not compress) from the vein (*blue arrow*; will compress). **(c)** U/S, Doppler mode, confirming pulsatile arterial blood flow through the RA (red, arterial; blue, venous). **(d)** U/S, longitudinal orientation, confirming that the guidewire (*white arrow*) is within the lumen of the RA origin. The *yellow arrow* indicates the RA puncture site.

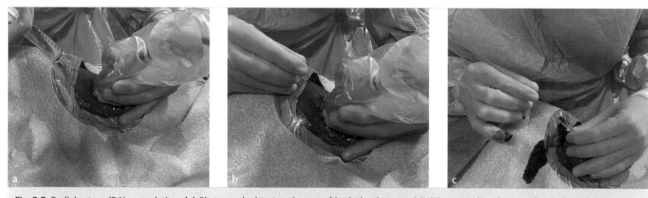

Fig. 2.5 Radial artery (RA) cannulation. **(a)** Photograph showing the use of bedside ultrasound (U/S) to visualize the RA. The probe is held perpendicular to the course of the RA. The use of a local injection of lidocaine is reserved for cases performed without the use of general anesthesia. **(b)** The RA is punctured with a needle until pulsatile arterial blood return is visualized. **(c)** The guidewire is gently advanced. If any resistance is encountered, we use fluoroscopy to ensure the guidewire is not selecting a side branch or deviates from the expected RA course.

- RA access-site complications often look very dramatic on angiography, but fortunately are very forgiving in most cases (▶ Fig. 2.11). Close attention to patency of distal pulses, limb temperature, and pain is needed to recognize compartment syndrome or critical limb ischemia.

- RA anatomical variants such as an RA loop or the presence of a radial recurrent artery (▶ Fig. 2.12) are commonly cited as reasons for RA access failure. Awareness of these normal variants and knowledge of specific techniques to manage them can help establish quick access in many such cases.

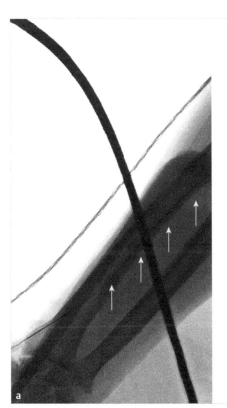
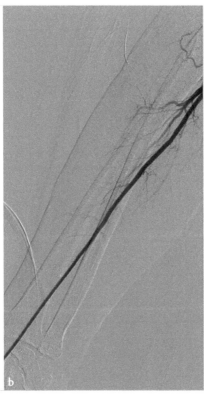

Fig. 2.6 Radial artery (RA) access with a sheath. **(a)** Fluoroscopy, confirming the course of the guidewire along the right RA (*arrows*). The radial sheath can be safely placed. **(b)** Digital subtraction angiography (DSA), RA injection, confirming successful placement of the sheath.

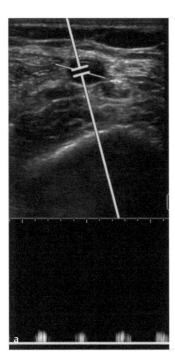
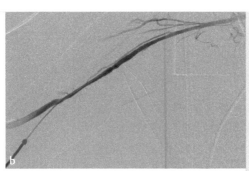
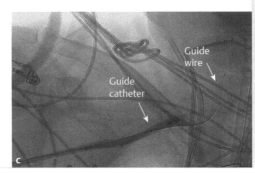

Fig. 2.7 Brachial artery access. **(a)** Ultrasound (U/S), transverse image, localizing the brachial artery (top half) and confirming pulsatile arterial blood flow (bottom half). **(b)** Digital subtraction angiography (DSA), brachial artery injection, showing regional vasospasm. The injection is performed via a 5F dilator (Cook Medical). Ten mg of verapamil was given through the dilator. A 6F sheath was exchanged for the dilator (not shown). **(c)** Angiography, unsubtracted view, showing a 0.071-inch guide catheter (*yellow arrow*; Benchmark [Penumbra]) and a 0.035-inch guidewire (*white arrow*; GlideWire [Terumo]).

Guide wire

Guide catheter

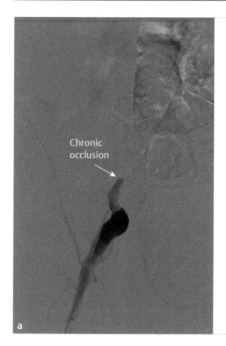

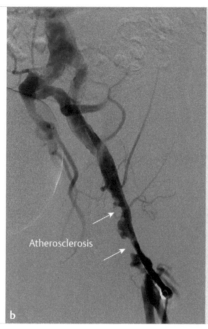

Fig. 2.8 Femoral artery (FA) atherosclerosis. **(a)** Digital subtraction angiography (DSA), right common FA injection, showing a chronic occlusion (*arrow*). The injection was performed using a 5F dilator. Often, failure of the microwire to advance further indicates the possibility of occlusion (or dissection); in such cases, using a dilator to perform DSA can be helpful. **(b)** DSA, left common FA, showing diffuse, severe atherosclerosis (*arrows*), precluding safe use of a percutaneous closure device.

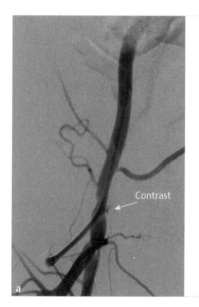

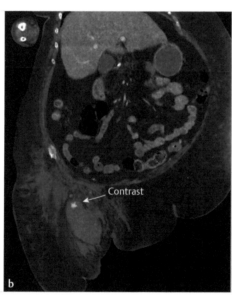

Fig. 2.9 Groin hematoma after femoral artery (FA) access. **(a)** Digital subtraction angiography (DSA), right common FA injection, showing placement of a 7F sheath above the common FA bifurcation and below the origin of the inferior epigastric artery. Given focal underlying stenosis, a closure device was not used and manual pressure was applied at the end of the case. A subtle area of contrast extravasation (*arrow*) was not initially appreciated. **(b)** Computed tomography (CT) of the abdomen and pelvis, showing a right groin hematoma with a small area of active contrast extravasation (*arrow*). The study was obtained after postprocedure groin checks showed an enlarging groin mass. Additional manual pressure was applied, and the therapeutic effect of the previous systemic heparinization was reversed with protamine.

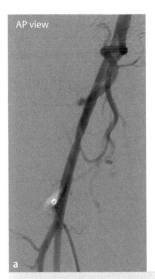
AP view

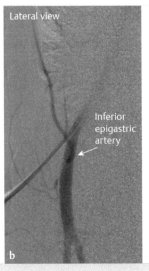
Lateral view

Inferior epigastric artery

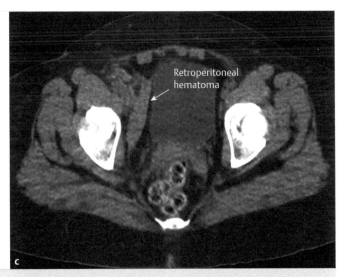
Retroperitoneal hematoma

Fig. 2.10 Retroperitoneal hematoma after femoral artery (FA) access. **(a)** Digital subtraction angiography (DSA), right common FA injection, anteroposterior (AP) view, showing what appears to be an optimal femoral sheath placement. No active contrast extravasation or signs of dissection or other vessel injury is seen. **(b)** DSA, right common FA injection, lateral view. Here, the femoral sheath entering above the origin of the inferior epigastric artery (*arrow*) is clearly seen. In such cases, there is a risk of retroperitoneal hematoma formation. **(c)** Computed tomography (CT) of the abdomen and pelvis, showing a small retroperitoneal hematoma (*arrow*). The CT was obtained after the patient complained of extensive back pain. Fortunately, repeat CT showed stable hematoma size, and no further intervention was required.

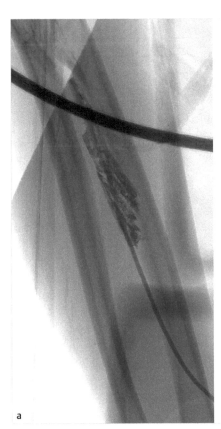

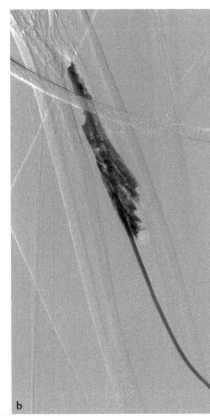

Fig. 2.11 Radial artery (RA) perforation. **(a)** Unsubtracted and **(b)** digital subtraction angiography (DSA), left RA injection, antero-posterior (AP) view, showing RA perforation with active contrast extravasation into the surrounding muscle. This likely occurred because the 0.018-inch guidewire selected a side branch of the RA. Angiographic assessment of the course of the guidewire is always necessary before sheath placement.

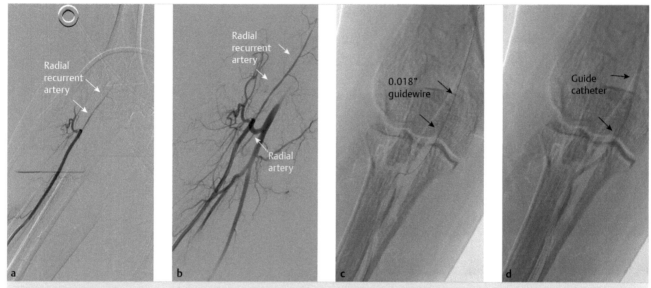

Fig. 2.12 Radial recurrent artery and its management during radial artery (RA) access. **(a)** Digital subtraction angiography (DSA), right RA injection, anteroposterior (AP) view, showing a glimpse of the proximal portion of the RA (*arrows*). In fact, this is the radial recurrent artery, which is the largest lateral branch of the RA in the forearm, arising close to its origin. If underrecognized, the guidewire and catheter can be navigated into this branch, causing its damage. **(b)** DSA, repeat RA injection with a large amount of contrast material and the guide catheter positioned more proximally, showing the true course of the proximal RA (*yellow arrow*). The *white arrows* point to the radial recurrent artery. **(c)** Roadmap, RA injection, showing a 0.018-inch guidewire (*arrows*; Aristotle [Scientia Vascular]) navigated into the brachial artery. **(d)** Roadmap, RA injection, showing a 0.071-inch guide catheter (*arrows*; Benchmark [Penumbra]) access. Placing this guide into the radial recurrent artery would likely result in its perforation and eventual failure to catheterize the brachial artery.

2.6 Cases with Videos and Images

2.6.1 Case 2.1 RA Loop

A patient with a suspected basilar artery occlusion is taken for emergent thrombectomy. Radial artery (RA) access is planned. This case illustrates the recognition and management of a RA loop discovered after performing the initial RA angiogram (▶ **Video 2.1**; ▶ Fig. 2.13, ▶ Fig. 2.14, ▶ Fig. 2.15).

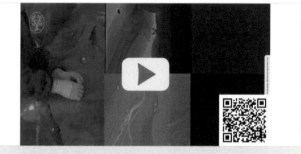

Video 2.1 Radial Artery Loop.

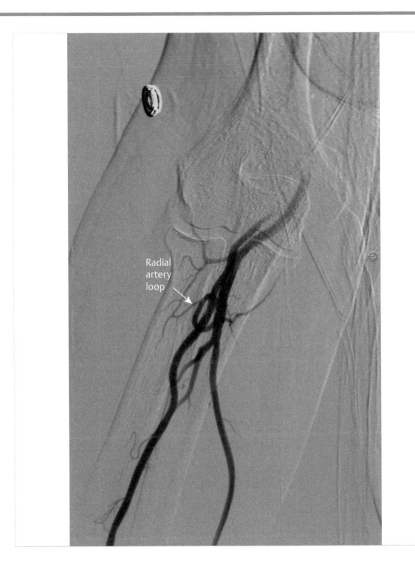

Radial
artery
loop

Fig. 2.13 Baseline digital subtraction angiography (DSA). Right radial artery (RA) injection, anteroposterior (AP) view, showing a loop of the proximal RA (*arrow*). Attempts to cross the loop with a 0.035-inch hydrophilic-coated guidewire (GlideWire [Terumo]) are unsuccessful (not shown).

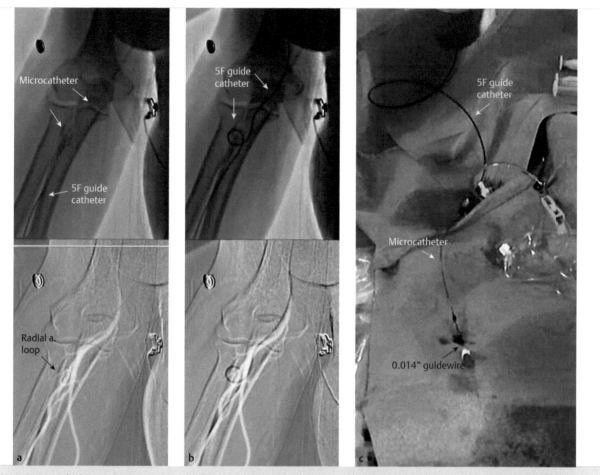

Fig. 2.14 Crossing the loop with a microcatheter. (a) Fluoroscopy (top image) and roadmap (bottom image), radial artery (RA) injection, showing delivery of a 0.025-inch microcatheter (*white arrows*; Velocity [Penumbra]) around the RA loop (*black arrow*). A 0.014-inch guidewire (Synchro [Stryker]) was used to cross the loop and help navigate the microcatheter (not shown). A 5F guide is positioned distal to the loop (*yellow arrow*). (b) Fluoroscopy (top image) and roadmap (bottom image), RA injection, showing the 5F guide (*yellow arrow*) now being navigated around the loop using microcatheter–guidewire support. (c) Photograph showing devices used to cross the RA loop. *White arrow*, 0.025-inch Velocity microcatheter (Penumbra); *black arrow*, 0.014-inch Synchro guidewire (Stryker) with a torque device attached to it; and *yellow arrow*, 5F guide catheter.

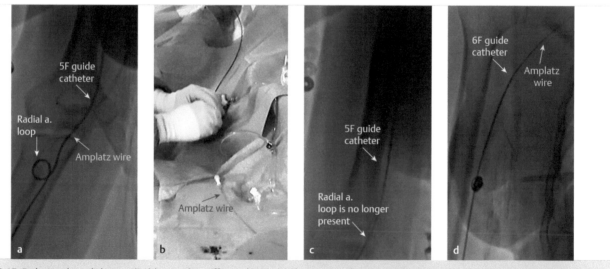

Fig. 2.15 Reducing the radial artery (RA) loop with a stiffer guidewire. (a) Fluoroscopy, showing a stiffer 0.035-inch Amplatz stainless steel guidewire (*green arrow*; Boston Scientific) being delivered through the 5F guide catheter (*yellow arrow*). The RA loop is still present (*white arrow*) because the most distal portion of the Amplatz wire is rather soft. (b) Photograph showing the operator advancing the Amplatz wire (*arrow*). (c) Fluoroscopy showing the RA loop being reduced (*white arrow*) as the Amplatz wire is advanced farther into the guide catheter (*yellow arrow*). (d) Fluoroscopy showing exchange for a large 6F 0.071-inch guide catheter (*yellow arrow*; Benchmark [Penumbra]). The *green arrow* points to the Amplatz wire. The guide catheter can now be easily navigated into the VA (not shown).

3 Challenging Access

General Description

Establishing arterial access and reaching the occlusion are key steps in the thrombectomy procedure. Carefully reviewing the patient's anatomy and selecting the optimal tools are critical for the ability to navigate an anatomically challenging arch and cervical tortuosity. Many failures or delays to establish successful reperfusion are directly related to suboptimal guide catheter access and selection of thrombectomy devices not suitable for certain anatomical variants. Here, we provide examples of common techniques that can help the operator to recognize and avoid such mistakes.

Keywords: aortic arch, carotid dissection tortuosity, triaxial

3.1 Anatomical and Imaging Aspects

- Computed tomography angiography (CTA) or magnetic resonance angiography (MRA) is extremely helpful in understanding the arch and great vessel anatomy before intervention.
- Classifying the arch type (▶ Fig. 3.1) and noting anatomical variations (▶ Fig. 3.2), ostial disease, tandem occlusions, or severe tortuosity help the operator choose the most appropriate access site (femoral vs. radial), guide catheter, support catheter, and guidewire.

3.2 Technique and Key Steps

- For aortic arch type II and III, we prefer using a VTK-type catheter such as a 5-French (F) VTK (Cook Medical). A stiffer 0.035-inch guidewire or 0.038-inch guidewire such as Stiff GlideWire (Terumo) can be used to "straighten" the arch, changing its configuration from type III to II, thus easing the delivery of a guide catheter (▶ Fig. 3.3).
- An additional wire ("buddy" wire) can be used for guide catheter support. We typically use a V18 guidewire (Boston Scientific), which is a 0.018-inch stainless steel wire. A buddy wire is commonly used when ostial or proximal lesions require treatment (▶ Fig. 3.4).
- When selecting guide catheter and thrombectomy devices, considerations include the location of tandem lesions and working length of the guide catheter, aspiration catheter, and microcatheter (▶ Fig. 3.5) to ensure that the target location can be successfully reached with the device.

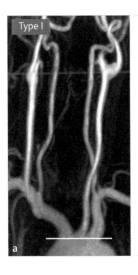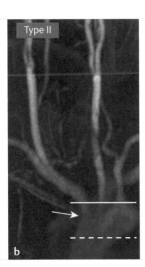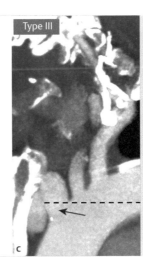

Fig. 3.1 Aortic arch classification. The origin of the brachiocephalic artery and level of the top of the aortic arch are used for classification. **(a)** Type I arch. Magnetic resonance angiography (MRA), coronal projection. All three great vessel origins are at the apex of the arch (*solid line*). Obtaining access in such cases is rather straightforward. **(b)** Type II arch. MRA, coronal projection. The takeoff of the brachiocephalic artery (*arrow*) is between outer (*solid line*) and inner curves (*dashed line*) of the arch. **(c)** Type III arch. Computed tomography angiography (CTA), coronal projection. This is the most challenging type of arch for access. The origin of the brachiocephalic artery (*arrow*) is at or below the level of the inner curve of the arch (*dashed line*).

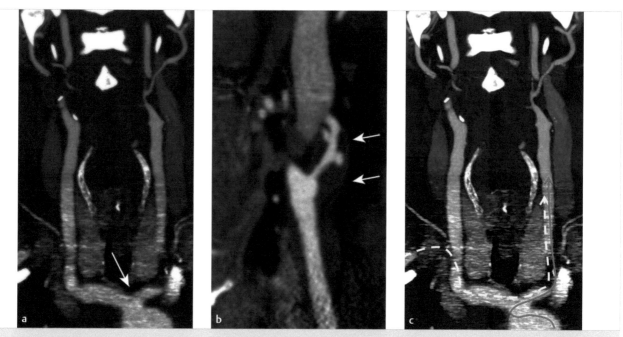

Fig. 3.2 Bovine arch. **(a)** The brachiocephalic artery and left common carotid artery (CCA) share a common origin (*arrow*), as shown on the computed tomography angiography (CTA). Note the sharp angle created by the left CCA. Transfemoral access in such cases can be rather challenging. Right radial access is often preferable, depending on the degree of the left CCA takeoff angle. **(b)** CTA, lateral view, showing a highly ulcerated plaque of the left internal carotid artery (ICA) origin (*arrows*). This plaque was the likely cause of the patient's tandem left middle cerebral artery (MCA) occlusion. **(c)** Planning access. Right radial artery access in this case is more ergonomic (*yellow dashed line*), minimizing the risk of the guidewire or catheter "jumping" and disturbing the plaque. Femoral access would require maneuvers to overcome sharp left CCA origin angulation (*red line*) to establish guide catheter access.

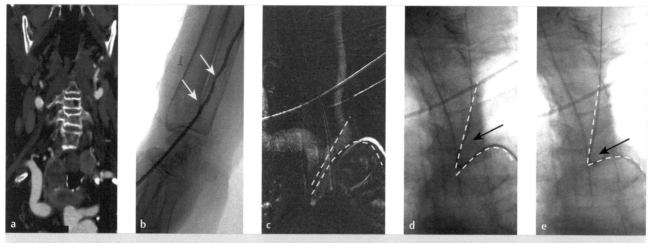

Fig. 3.3 Changing the left common carotid artery (CCA) angle with a stiff guidewire. **(a)** Computed tomography angiography (CTA), coronal view, demonstrating a bovine arch. Left middle cerebral artery (MCA) thrombectomy is planned. Radial artery access was attempted first but was unsuccessful due to radial artery vasospasm resistant to medical treatment. **(b)** Right radial artery injection showing severe vasospasm precluding further advancement of the radial sheath. Transfemoral access was attempted next. **(c)** Roadmap, anteroposterior (AP) projection, showing bovine arch. Transfemoral access into the left internal carotid artery (ICA) in this case is rather challenging due to the acute arch-left common carotid artery (CCA) angle (*dashed yellow lines*). Access into the left ICA is being pursued. A stiff 0.038-inch GlideWire (Terumo) is used for access in this case. **(d,e)** Fluoroscopy, AP views, showing gradual widening of the angle of the arch and left CCA (indicated by *dashed yellow lines*) by advancing the guide catheter more distally. The arrow in each images points to the tip of the 5F VTK catheter (Cook Medical) used to facilitate access into the left CCA.

3.3 Pearls and Pitfalls

- Local vasospasm, mainly due to guide catheter manipulation, is frequently encountered during thrombectomy procedures. Although it creates flow arrest (similar to the use of a balloon guide catheter [BGC]), early recognition of this adverse event and its correction by withdrawing the catheter more proximally and, depending on the degree of spasm, possibly administering local calcium channel blockers are advised. If untreated,

vasospasm can interfere with further advancement of the guide or intermediate catheter (▶ Fig. 3.6). Severe vasospasm can also predispose to clot formation due to prolonged flow arrest, because systemic heparinization is not typically administered during thrombectomy cases (▶ Fig. 3.7).
- Underlying fibromuscular dysplasia should alert the interventionist about the possibility of iatrogenic dissection. Advancing a guide or an intermediate catheter or withdrawing a stent retriever (SR) should be performed with extra caution (▶ Fig. 3.8).

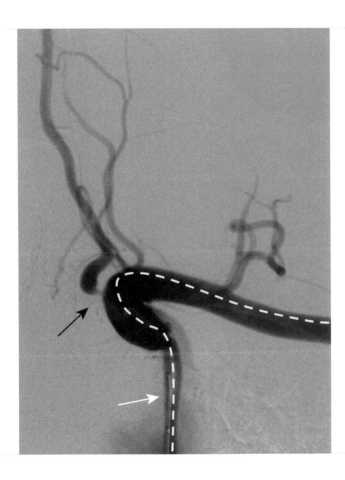

Fig. 3.4 Using a "buddy" wire. Digital subtraction angiogram (DSA), anteroposterior (AP) view, left subclavian artery injection showing severe vertebral artery origin stenosis (*black arrow*). Left radial access would be preferable in this case but could not be obtained. A guide catheter (0.087-inch 6F shuttle [Cook Medical]) is positioned just barely beyond the origin of the left subclavian artery. To prevent guide catheter herniation, a V18 guidewire (Boston Scientific) will be introduced through the guide catheter and into the left subclavian artery (*dashed line*) before the operator addresses the vertebral artery (VA) stenosis lesion. A balloon-mounted stent can be seen being delivered through the guide catheter (*white arrow*).

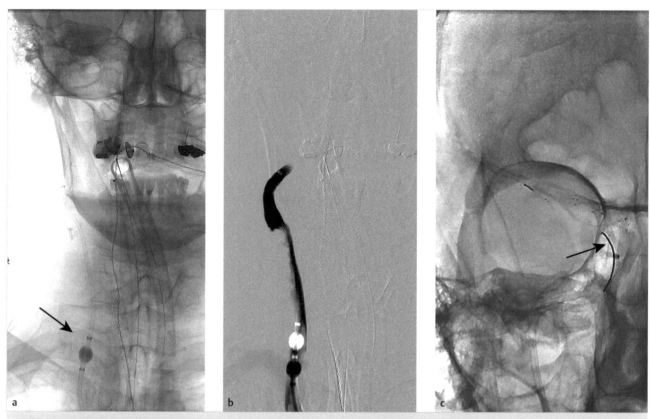

Fig. 3.5 Accounting for catheter length during thrombectomy. **(a)** Fluoroscopy, anteroposterior (AP) view, showing a balloon guide catheter (BGC) (Walrus, Q'Apel Medical) positioned in the origin of the right common carotid artery (CCA) (*arrow*). **(b)** Right CCA injection, AP view, showing a large clot burden within the right CCA. Thus, the guide catheter is not advanced any farther, and thrombectomy is pursued using a long aspiration catheter and a stent receiver (SR). **(c)** Fluoroscopy, AP projection, showing an SR (EmboTrap, Cerenovus) placed into the M1 segment with the assistance of a Sofia Plus aspiration catheter (MicroVention). A 131-cm Sofia Plus (*arrow*) and 90-cm Walrus are chosen for this case to ensure that the aspiration catheter can reach the M1 segment even with such a "low" position of the BGC.

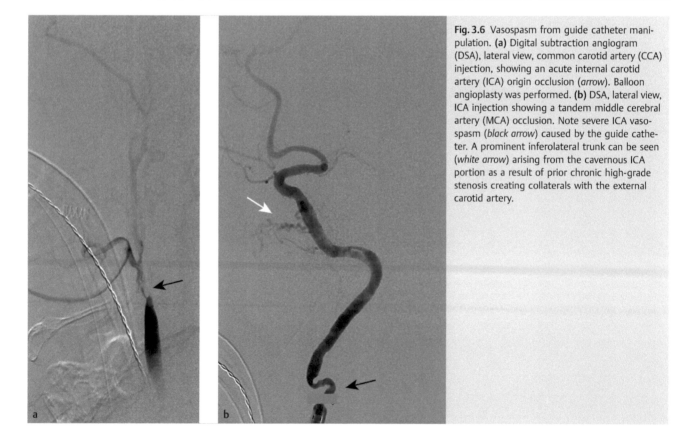

Fig. 3.6 Vasospasm from guide catheter manipulation. **(a)** Digital subtraction angiogram (DSA), lateral view, common carotid artery (CCA) injection, showing an acute internal carotid artery (ICA) origin occlusion (*arrow*). Balloon angioplasty was performed. **(b)** DSA, lateral view, ICA injection showing a tandem middle cerebral artery (MCA) occlusion. Note severe ICA vasospasm (*black arrow*) caused by the guide catheter. A prominent inferolateral trunk can be seen (*white arrow*) arising from the cavernous ICA portion as a result of prior chronic high-grade stenosis creating collaterals with the external carotid artery.

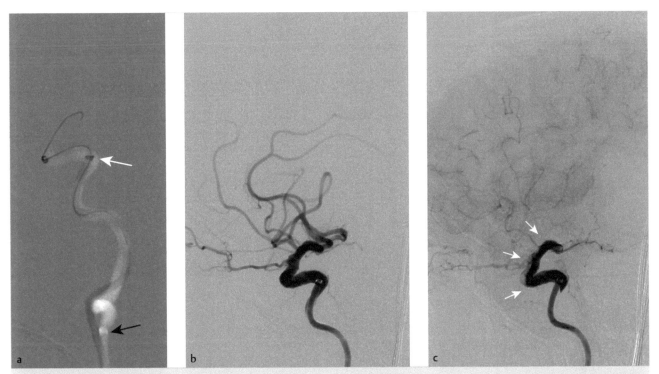

Fig. 3.7 Vasospasm causing flow arrest. **(a)** Fluoroscopy, lateral view, internal carotid artery (ICA) injection. Note vasospasm (*black arrow*) at the initial level of the 0.088-inch guide catheter (Zoom 88 [Imperative Care]). The operator chose to proceed with further advancement of the guide catheter into the cavernous segment (*white arrow*) without addressing the vasospasm first. **(b)** Right ICA injection, lateral view, confirming middle cerebral artery (MCA) occlusion. **(c)** Right ICA injection, capillary phase, shows persistent stasis of contrast material within the ICA intracranially (*arrows*) as a result of proximal flow arrest caused by ICA spasm around the guide catheter. This prompted withdrawal of the guide catheter, administration of calcium channel blockers, and re-establishing guide catheter access.

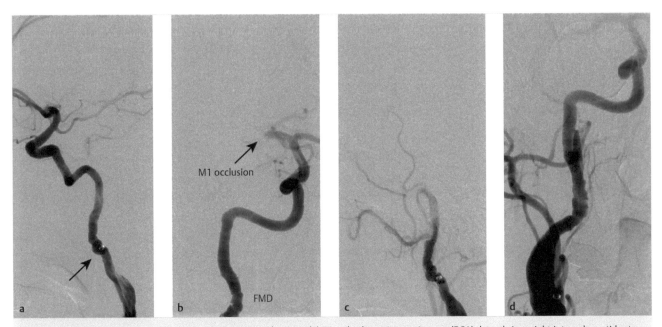

Fig. 3.8 Fibromuscular dysplasia (FMD) complicating arterial access. **(a)** Digital subtraction angiogram (DSA), lateral view, right internal carotid artery (ICA) injection, showing middle cerebral artery (MCA) occlusion. Note the diseased appearance of the cervical ICA segment near the guide catheter tip (*arrow*). **(b)** DSA, anteroposterior (AP) view, demonstrating local FMD of the distal cervical ICA. MCA M1 occlusion is present (*arrow*). **(c)** DSA, lateral view, showing complete occlusion of the ICA as a result of dissection caused by attempts to advance the guide catheter through the arterial segment with underlying FMD. **(d)** DSA, anteroposterior (AP) view, showing repaired ICA dissection using an intracranial stent (4.5 mm × 30 mm Neuroform Atlas [Styker]).

3.4 Cases with Videos and Images

3.4.1 Case 3.1 Balloon Guide Catheter Anchoring Technique

A case of left middle cerebral artery (MCA) occlusion with tortuous carotid artery access based on craniocervical computed tomography angiography (CTA) results. A balloon guide catheter (BGC) is used in this case to establish access into the left internal carotid artery (ICA) to pursue thrombectomy (▶ **Video 3.1**; ▶ Fig. 3.9, ▶ Fig. 3.10, ▶ Fig. 3.11, ▶ Fig. 3.12, ▶ Fig. 3.13).

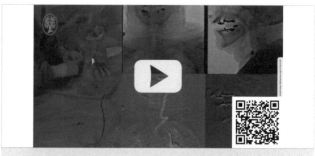

Video 3.1 Balloon Guide Catheter Anchoring Technique.

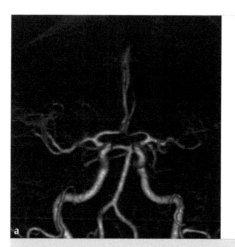
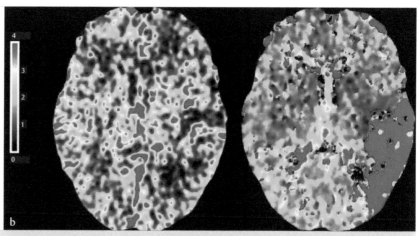

Fig. 3.9 Baseline noninvasive imaging. **(a)** Computed tomography angiography (CTA), coronal view, showing left middle cerebral artery (MCA) occlusion. **(b)** CT perfusion image showing preserved volume (image on left) but delayed flow (image on right) in the corresponding left MCA territory.

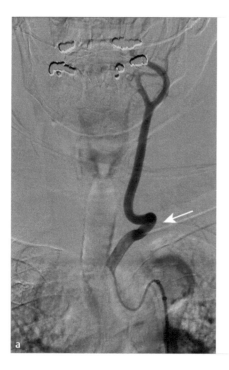
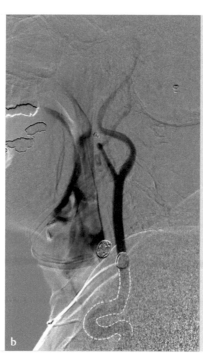

Fig. 3.10 Left common carotid artery (CCA) tortuosity. Digital subtraction angiogram (DSA): **(a)** anteroposterior (AP) and **(b)** lateral views, showing tortuosity of the left CCA proximally (*arrow*). Sharp angulation of the CCA on the lateral projection is highlighted with *dashed lines*.

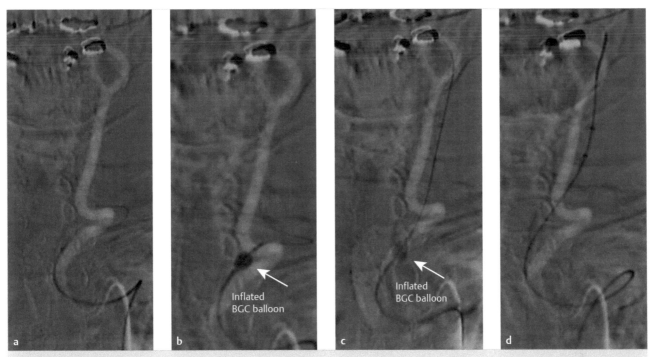

Fig. 3.11 Left common carotid artery (CCA) access with balloon guide catheter. **(a–d)** Anteroposterior (AP) views, roadmaps, showing guide catheter stability achieved with balloon inflation (*white arrow*). This allows access with the guidewire into the left internal carotid artery (ICA) without causing guide herniation into the arch.

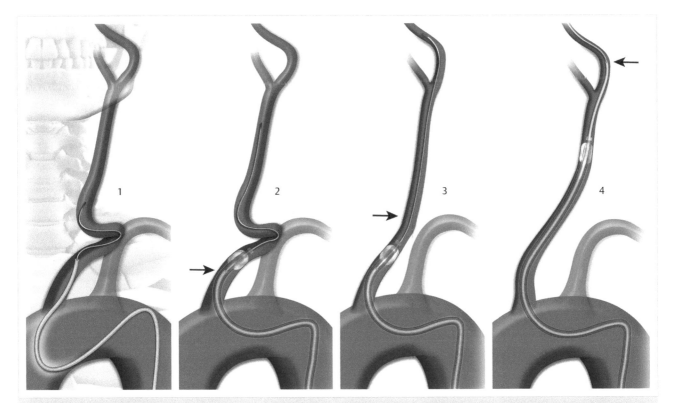

Fig. 3.12 Artist's illustration of the balloon-anchoring technique. Key steps of using a balloon guide catheter (BGC) are illustrated here. Step 1—A "traditional" approach of using a Simmons-type or VTK-type catheter fails to provide adequate support for a guidewire to access the tortuous anatomy. Step 2—Inflating the balloon creates a balloon-type anchor (*arrow*), locking the guide in place. Step 3—The stability achieved with balloon inflation allows further advancement of the guidewire, straightening the unfavorable anatomical tortuosity (*arrow*). Step 4—The guide and aspiration catheters can now be navigated into the distal location (*arrow*). (© Thieme/Jennifer Pryll)

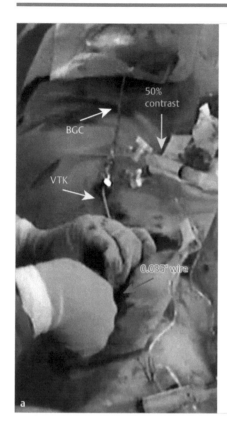
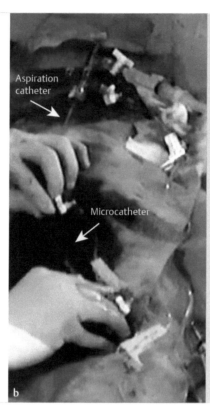

Fig. 3.13 Procedural catheter setup for guide catheter access and thrombectomy. **(a)** Procedural photograph showing balloon guide catheter (BGC) (*white arrow*) with the balloon inflated using a syringe filled with 50% contrast material (*green arrow*). The operator is advancing a 0.035-inch guidewire (*red arrow*) with the support of a VTK-type catheter (*yellow arrow*). **(b)** Photograph showing preparation for thrombectomy. An intermediate catheter (*white arrow*, 6F Sofia [MicroVention]) and 0.025-inch microcatheter (*yellow arrow*, Velocity [Penumbra]) are used.

3.4.2 Case 3.2 ICA Loop and "Soft" Long Guide Sheath

This case illustrates guide catheter access in a patient with tortuous common carotid artery (CCA) and internal carotid artery (ICA) anatomy including a 360-degree cervical ICA loop. The patient presented with sudden onset of right hemispheric stroke syndrome caused by a proximal right middle cerebral artery (MCA) occlusion (▶ **Video 3.2**, ▶ Fig. 3.14, ▶ Fig. 3.15, ▶ Fig. 3.16, ▶ Fig. 3.17, ▶ Fig. 3.18, ▶ Fig. 3.19).

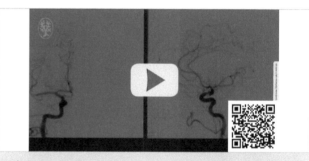

Video 3.2 Internal Carotid Artery Loop and "Soft" Long Guide Sheath.

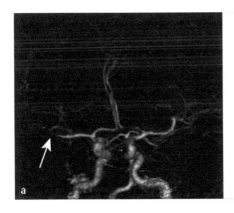

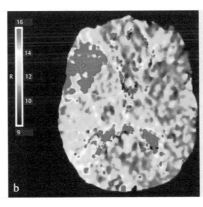

Fig. 3.14 Baseline noninvasive imaging. (a) Computed tomography angiography (CTA) showing a distal middle cerebral artery (MCA) M1 occlusion (*arrow*). (b) Computed tomography (CT) perfusion map with a corresponding perfusion deficit in the right MCA territory.

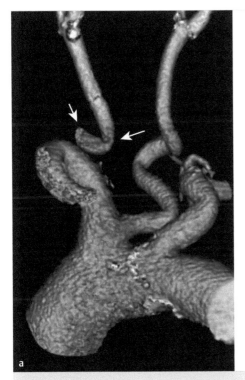

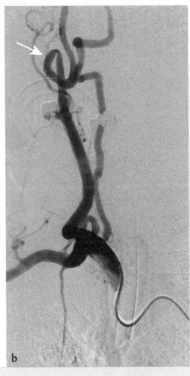

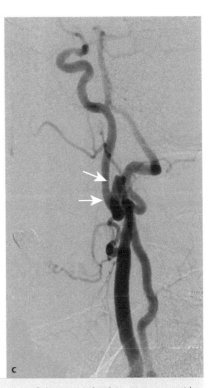

Fig. 3.15 Carotid artery tortuosity. (a) Computed tomography angiography (CTA) showing tortuous course of the proximal right common carotid artery (CCA) (*arrows*). Digital subtraction angiogram (DSA) (b). Anteroposterior (AP) and (c) lateral views showing severe tortuosity of the cervical right internal carotid artery (ICA) with a 360-degree loop (*arrows*).

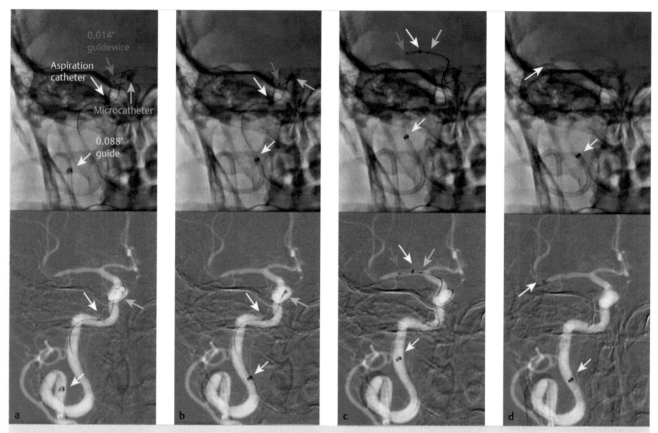

Fig. 3.16 Delivery of guide and aspiration catheters. **(a–d)** Anteroposterior (AP) views, live fluoroscopy (top images) with corresponding roadmaps (bottom images), showing gradual delivery of guide catheter (*yellow arrow*, Zoom 88 [Imperative Care]) around the 360-degree loop and aspiration catheter (*white arrow*, 6F Sofia Plus [MicroVention]) at the M1 occlusion site. Note that the guidewire (*red arrow*) and microcatheter (*green arrow*) never traverse the clot. The guide catheter is first kept proximal to the 360-degree loop. Once the aspiration catheter is positioned distally, the guide is pushed forward around the 360-degree cervical loop.

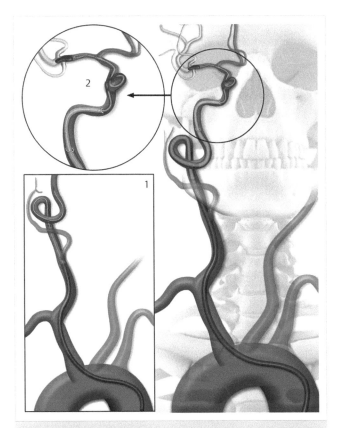

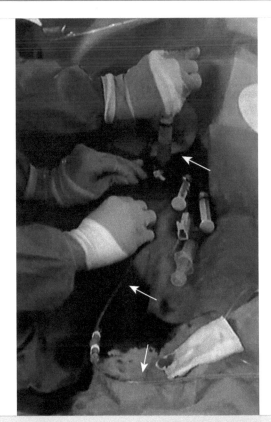

Fig. 3.17 Artist's illustration showing guide access and aspiration catheter delivery. The guide catheter is initially placed proximal to the 360-degree loop to avoid getting a dissection (1). Using a triaxial approach over the guidewire-microcatheter-aspiration catheter, the guide catheter can now be safely advanced around the 360-degree loop without distorting this challenging anatomy. (2) The aspiration catheter is then advanced to face the M1 clot. (© Thieme/Jennifer Pryll)

Fig. 3.18 Aspiration thrombectomy. Procedural photograph showing aspiration tubing (*white arrows*) connected to the aspiration catheter. Minimal blood return can be seen inside the tubing, indicating that the catheter lumen is completely occupied by clot. While the catheter is slowly withdrawn, additional aspiration is applied via a syringe through the guide catheter (*yellow arrow*).

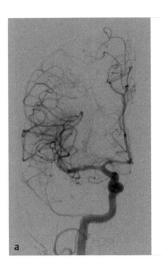
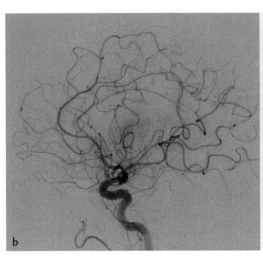

Fig. 3.19 Postaspiration angiography. **(a)** Antero-posterior (AP) and **(b)** lateral views showing thrombolysis in cerebral infarction grade 3 reperfusion with first-pass effect.

4 Common Carotid Artery Occlusion

General Description

Most acute ischemic stroke (AIS) as a result of carotid artery disease involves the internal carotid artery (ICA). Total occlusion or severe stenosis of the common carotid artery (CCA) as a cause of AIS is relatively rare. Radiographically, the disease can involve the CCA segment only or extend more distally into the ICA. Similar to the management of the ICA in the setting of AIS, the decision to proceed with emergent stenting of the CCA depends on the severity of the stenosis or the presence of complete occlusion, whether tandem intracranial occlusion is present, and the amount of the stroke burden (size of the ischemic core).

Keywords: Carotid stent, common carotid artery, covered stent

4.1 Anatomical and Imaging Aspects

- Atherosclerosis is the most common cause of CCA occlusion (▶ Fig. 4.1). Other potential etiologies may include a dissection (often including the aortic arch), Takayasu arteritis, massive embolus (infectious, hypercoagulable state (▶ Fig. 4.2), or cardioembolic), or radiation-induced changes.

- Computed tomography angiography (CTA) or magnetic resonance angiography (MRA) should include the aortic arch in order to accurately evaluate the status of the CCA from its origin to the carotid bulb. If noninvasive imaging studies are insufficient for depicting the arch and CCA origins, an aortic arch injection can be performed during catheter angiography (▶ Fig. 4.3).

- Positioning a guide catheter near the CCA origin, especially for a left CCA lesion, can be challenging. Using a second guide wire (buddy-wire), such as a V18 (Boston Scientific) placed into the right subclavian artery can improve the success rate of carotid cannulation with a guide catheter.

4.2 Carotid Stent Selection

- A large parent vessel diameter (the CCA diameter is often greater in comparison to the cervical ICA diameter) and lack of stable guide catheter access, especially in lesions involving the CCA origin, can be overcome by using covered stents. Covered stents (e.g., iCast [Atrium] or Viabahn [Cook]) require a large-bore guide catheter diameter (such as a 7–8 French [F] long sheath) and 0.035-inch guidewire support (such as a 0.035-inch stiff Amplatz guidewire [Cook]). Extreme caution is needed when placing a covered

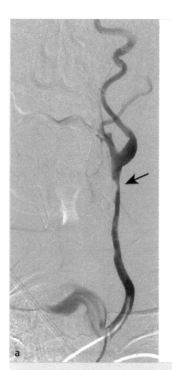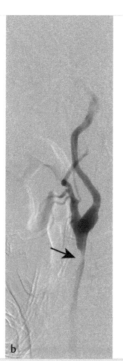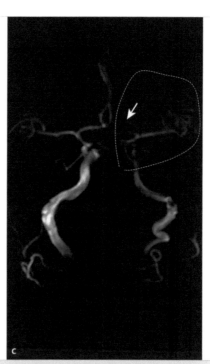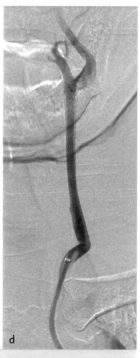

Fig. 4.1 Isolated flow-limiting stenosis of the common carotid artery (CCA) secondary to atherosclerosis treated with stenting. **(a)** Cervical digital subtraction angiogram (DSA), anteroposterior (AP) view, showing severe isolated stenosis of the distal CCA (*arrow*) from a long atherosclerotic plaque. **(b)** Near-complete occlusion of the distal CCA is best appreciated on this cervical DSA, lateral view (*arrow*). **(c)** Magnetic resonance angiography (MRA) demonstrating the flow-limiting nature of CCA stenosis, with diminished opacification of the left CCA territory intracranially (*outlined area*). Note the severely hypoplastic left A1 segment (*arrow*), explaining the lack of collateral flow. **(d)** Cervical DSA showing restored patency of the CCA after stenting.

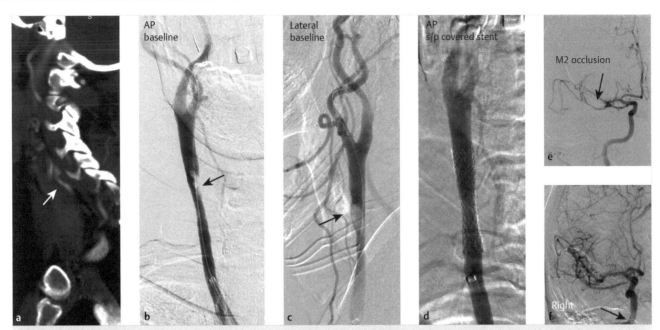

Fig. 4.2 Intraluminal thrombus of the right common carotid artery (CCA) and tandem occlusion of the M2 segment of the middle cerebral artery (MCA). **(a)** Cervical computed tomography angiography (CTA) showing a filling defect within the right CCA (*arrow*) representing a thrombus. This patient had a known active malignancy (hypercoagulable state) that resulted in intraluminal CCA thrombus with distal embolization into the MCA branches. **(b)** Digital subtraction angiogram (DSA), anteroposterior (AP) view, showing the thrombus (*arrow*). **(c)** DSA, lateral view. The thrombus occupies nearly the entire lumen of the CCA on this projection (*arrow*). **(d)** DSA, AP view, poststenting. A stent was used to "secure" the thrombus. Given the massive thrombus burden, attempts at removal could result in further embolization of downstream intracranial vessels. Once secured with the stent, the guide catheter can be carefully brought through the stent for optimal access to perform intracranial thrombectomy. Selecting a covered stent, rather than a traditional laser-cut or braided carotid stent, ensures that no embolic material escapes through the struts of the stent (so-called "cheese-grating" effect). **(e)** DSA, intracranial view, showing tandem M2 MCA occlusion (*arrow*). **(f)** DSA, intracranial view, post-thrombectomy. A thrombolysis in cerebral infarction (TICI) 2b score was achieved after several aspiration thrombectomy attempts. The *arrow* points to the tip of the guide catheter.

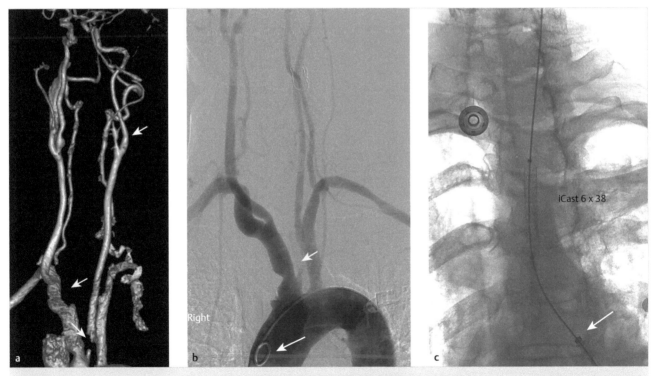

Fig. 4.3 Left common carotid artery (CCA) origin near-occlusion in a patient with a fluctuating degree of right-sided weakness. **(a)** Cervical computed tomography angiography (CTA) showing no significant left ICA stenosis (*white arrow*) that would explain the symptoms. CTA of the head was also unremarkable (not shown). However, the origins of the CCA were poorly visualized on the cervical CTA (*yellow arrows*), prompting emergent catheter angiography. **(b)** Digital subtraction angiogram (DSA), aortic arch run, using a 5F pigtail catheter (Merit Medical; *white arrow*). Note near-complete occlusion of the left CCA origin (*yellow arrows*), explaining the ongoing left hemispheric ischemia. **(c)** Fluoroscopy, anteroposterior (AP) view, showing emergent stenting using an iCast covered stent (Atrium). The arrow points to the 7F long sheath in the arch that was used to deliver the stent.

stent near the right CCA origin to ensure patency of the right subclavian artery.

- Because most large carotid stents or peripheral covered stents are rather rigid, we prefer using guide catheter sheaths capable of providing adequate support, such as 6–7F inner diameter Cook shuttle (Cook Medical) or Pinnacle Destination (Terumo) sheaths.

4.3 Pearls and Pitfalls

- Depending on the location of the CCA lesion and type of stent used, the use of embolic protection may not be feasible. For example, the use of a covered stent will preclude the use of a balloon guide catheter (BGC; "proximal" protection) as most covered stents require 7–8F inner diameter sheath access.
- Covered stents are highly thrombogenic, necessitating close adherence to dual antiplatelet therapy.
- In cases of tandem intracranial occlusion, once the CCA lesion is repaired, placement of an alternative longer and softer "neuro" guide catheter may be necessary for optimal access for intracranial thrombectomy.

4.4 Cases with Videos and Images

4.4.1 Case 4.1 Covered Stents in CCA Origin Occlusion

A patient with a fluctuating degree of right hemiparesis was found to have severe left common carotid artery (CCA) origin

stenosis. Pertinent medical history was significant for previous stenting of the brachiocephalic artery. Emergent stenting was planned (▸ **Video 4.1;** ▸ Fig. 4.4, ▸ Fig. 4.5, ▸ Fig. 4.6, ▸ Fig. 4.7).

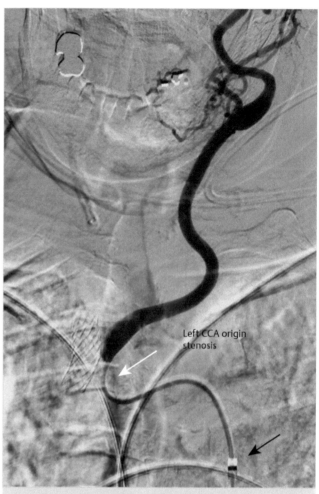

Fig. 4.4 Baseline digital subtraction angiogram (DSA) showing access into the left common carotid artery (CCA). VTK catheter (Cook; *white arrow*) is used to cross the area of left CCA stenosis just above the aortic arch. Such rather aggressive maneuvers are often needed because the left CCA origin lesions are particularly challenging to access. An 8F guide catheter is shown (*black arrow*).

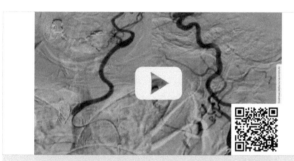

Video 4.1 Covered Stents in Common Carotid Artery Origin Occlusion.

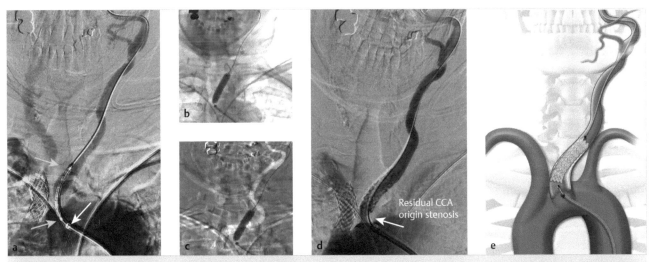

Fig. 4.5 Access through the lesion and stent placement. **(a)** Digital subtraction angiogram (DSA), intraprocedural view. Once access is obtained, with straightening of the carotid artery, the guide catheter (*white arrow*) is brought close to the lesion and a Viabahn covered stent (*yellow arrows*) is delivered. **(b)** Fluoroscopy and **(c)** roadmap showing balloon inflation with minimal overhang in the aortic arch. **(d)** DSA following placement of the first stent. There is no stent overhang into the aortic arch; however, there is some proximal stenosis that needs to be addressed (*arrow*). **(e)** Artist's illustration showing lack of adequate coverage of the CCA origin lesion by the most proximal part of the stent. (**e**: © Thieme/Jennifer Pryll)

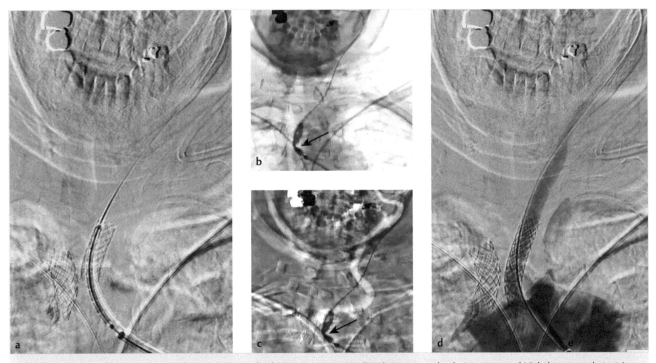

Fig. 4.6 Placement of a second covered stent. **(a)** Digital subtraction angiogram (DSA), intraprocedural view. A second Viabahn covered stent is brought, which will interlock with the first stent. **(b)** Fluoroscopy and **(c)** roadmap showing inflation of the second stent balloon once sufficient overlap between the two devices is achieved. The *arrows* indicate a "balloon waist" corresponding to the most severe area of stenosis. Note the significant straightening of the common carotid artery (CCA) caused by the stiff guidewire, best appreciated on the roadmap image. **(d)** DSA, postprocedural view. Patency of the left CCA origin is achieved.

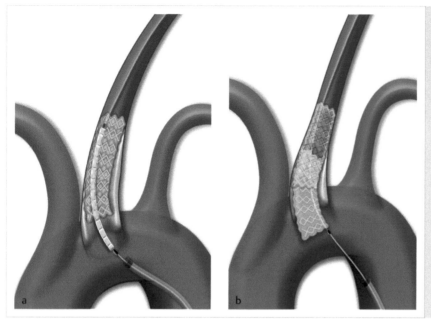

Fig. 4.7 Artist's illustration of placing a second covered stent to correct residual common carotid artery (CCA) origin stenosis. (a) A second stent is placed to allow interlocking of the two stents. (b) The second stent is deployed. The CCA origin stenosis is now completely covered. (© Thieme/ Jennifer Pryll)

4.4.2 Case 4.2 Common Carotid Artery Occlusion with a Long Lesion: A Two-Stent Construct

A patient is admitted with acute ischemic stroke with profound neurologic deficits: left hemiparesis, right gaze deviation, and neglect. Imaging in the emergency department reveals possible occlusion of the entire right carotid artery (▶ Video 4.2; ▶ Fig. 4.8, ▶ Fig. 4.9, ▶ Fig. 4.10, ▶ Fig. 4.11, ▶ Fig. 4.12, ▶ Fig. 4.13).

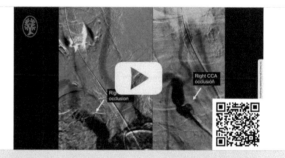

Video 4.2 Common Carotid Artery Occlusion with a Long Lesion: A Two-Stent Construct.

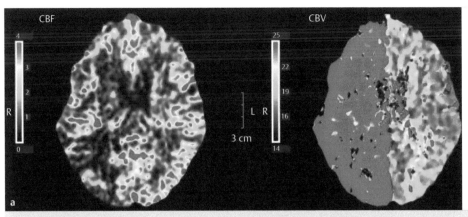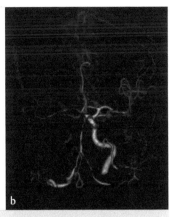

Fig. 4.8 Baseline imaging obtained on patient's presentation to the emergency department. **(a)** Reduced cerebral blood flow (CBF) (left) and increased cerebral blood volume (CBV) (right) within the entire right hemisphere can be seen. **(b)** Computed tomography angiography (CTA) three-dimensional (3D) reconstruction shows lack of opacification of the right internal carotid artery (ICA) and its branches.

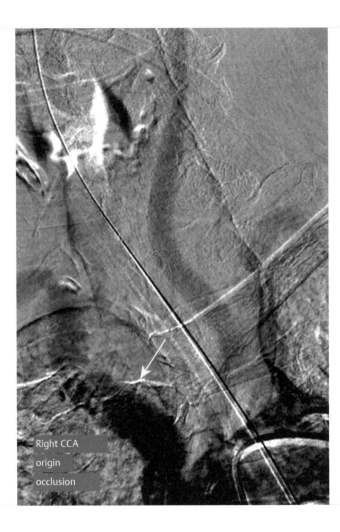

Right CCA origin occlusion

Fig. 4.9 Baseline digital subtraction angiogram (DSA). Anteroposterior (AP) view, aortic arch injection, showing a stump at the right common carotid artery (CCA) origin (*arrow*), confirming its complete occlusion.

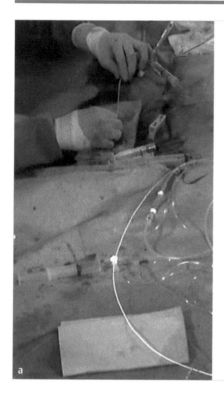

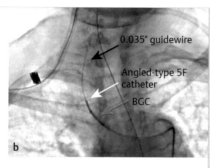

0.035" guidewire

Angled-type 5F catheter

BGC

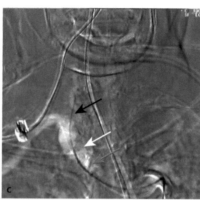

Fig. 4.10 Establishing access into the right common carotid artery (CCA). **(a)** A balloon guide catheter (BGC) (Walrus; Q'Apel Medical) is delivered over an angled-type catheter and a 0.035-inch guidewire system. The arrow points to the three-way stopcock and 1 mL and 10 mL syringes used to prepare the balloon on the guide catheter. **(b)** Fluoroscopy and **(c)** roadmap showing BGC delivery (*red arrow*) over an angled-type catheter (*white arrow*) and a 0.035-inch guidewire (*black arrow*).

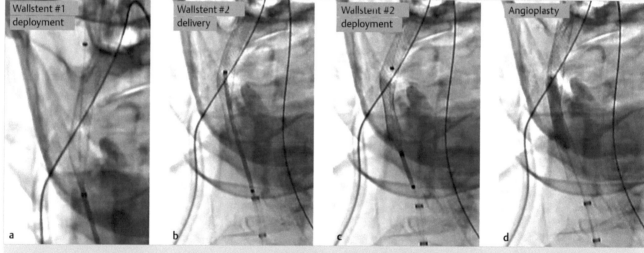

Wallstent #1 deployment

Wallstent #2 delivery

Wallstent #2 deployment

Angioplasty

Fig. 4.11 Delivery and placement of carotid stents under fluoroscopy. **(a)** Fluoroscopy showing delivery and partial deployment of the first carotid stent (Wallstent, Boston Scientific). **(b)** Fluoroscopy showing Wallstent fully deployed. Delivery of the second Wallstent is now performed to cover the more proximal area of the common carotid artery (CCA). **(c)** The second Wallstent is being deployed more proximally. **(d)** Angioplasty using an Aviator balloon (CardinalHealth) is performed at the maximal area of stenosis to ensure that the two stents adequately interlock with each other.

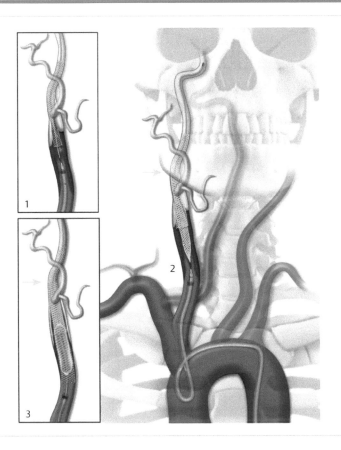

Fig. 4.12 Artist's illustration showing delivery and placement of two carotid stents. In step 1, the first carotid stent (*green color*) is delivered and deployed more distally. In step 2, the second carotid stent (*turquoise color*) is deployed to cover a more proximal area of stenosis, where a superimposed fresh clot can be seen. Finally, angioplasty is performed in step 3 to ensure optimal wall apposition of the two stents at their overlapping regions. (© Thieme/Jennifer Pryll)

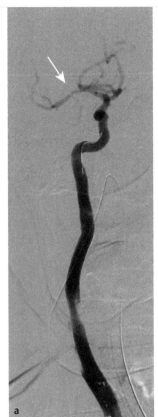

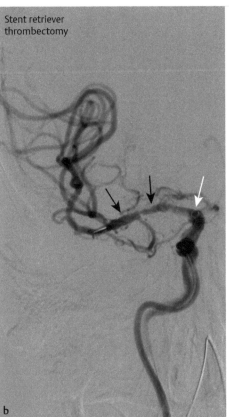

Stent retriever thrombectomy

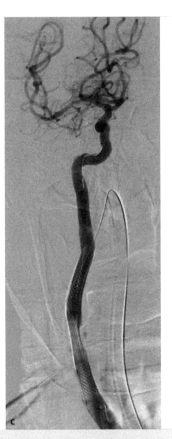

Fig. 4.13 Thrombectomy of tandem intracranial occlusion. **(a)** Digital subtraction angiogram (DSA), anteroposterior (AP) view showing restored patency of the right common carotid artery (CCA) after placement of two carotid stents. Downstream proximal middle cerebral artery (MCA) occlusion is present (*arrow*). **(b)** DSA, intraprocedural injection through the intermediate catheter (*white arrow*). A stent retriever (EmboTrap, Cerenovus) is seen deployed at the site of the right MCA M1–2 occlusion (*black arrows*). A temporary "endovascular bypass" is achieved from the radial force generated by the stent retriever device, allowing partial restoration of blood flow. **(c)** Post-thrombectomy DSA, right internal carotid artery (ICA) injection. Patency of the right MCA territory is achieved.

4.4.3 Case 4.3 Covered Stent Placement Through Brachial Access for Brachiocephalic Artery Occlusion

This patient presented with symptoms suggestive of an acute posterior circulation stroke. Noninvasive imaging was suggestive of a brachiocephalic artery occlusion. The brachial artery was chosen for access in this case (▶ **Video 4.3**; ▶ Fig. 4.14, ▶ Fig. 4.15, ▶ Fig. 4.16, ▶ Fig. 4.17, ▶ Fig. 4.18).

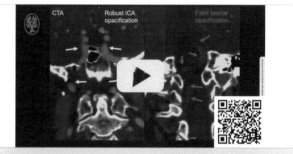

Video 4.3 Covered Stent Placement Through Brachial Access for Brachiocephalic Artery Occlusion.

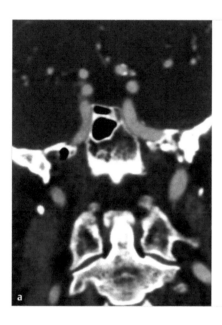
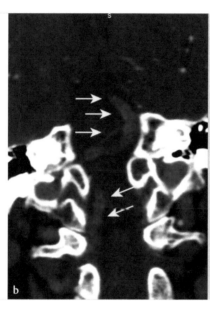

Fig. 4.14 Craniocervical computed tomography angiography (CTA) performed in the emergency department. **(a)** Robust opacification of both internal carotid arteries (ICAs) is seen. **(b)** Very faint contrast opacification is apparent within the right vertebral artery and the basilar artery (*arrows*).

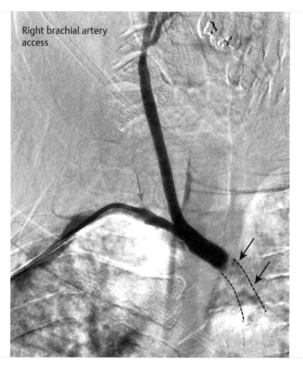

Fig. 4.15 Digital subtraction angiogram (DSA) performed via right brachial access. The *black arrows* and *broken line* point to the location of the occluded right brachiocephalic artery. A diagnostic catheter (*red arrow*) is shown.

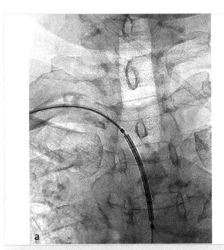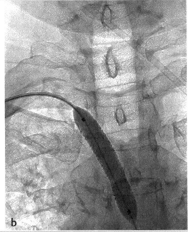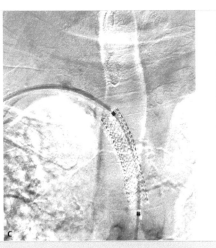

Fig. 4.16 Delivery and placement of a balloon-mounted covered stent. **(a)** Intraprocedural fluoroscopy, anteroposterior (AP) view, showing the position of the stent before deployment. A 0.035-inch guidewire is placed into the aortic arch for support. Anatomical landmarks are used to ensure optimal positioning of the stent to ensure that the origins of the right common carotid artery (CCA) and subclavian artery are not compromised during stent deployment. **(b)** Intraprocedural fluoroscopy showing inflation of the balloon and stent deployment. **(c)** Intraprocedural fluoroscopy showing the fully deployed stent.

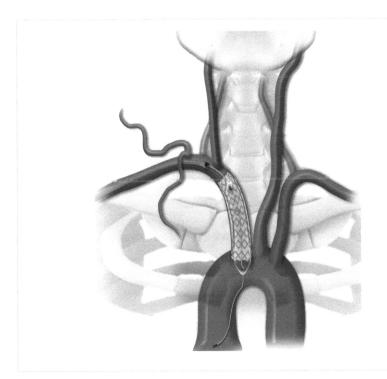

Fig. 4.17 Artist's illustration showing stenting of the brachiocephalic artery. Note exact location of the stent, sparing the origins of the right subclavian artery and common carotid artery (CCA). This is critical, because an incorrectly deployed covered stent can inadvertently cover the origin of these two main brachiocephalic artery branches. (© Thieme/Jennifer Pryll)

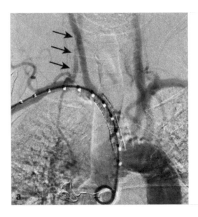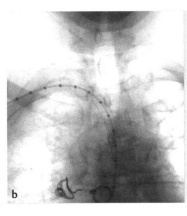

Fig. 4.18 Digital subtraction angiogram (DSA) after stent placement. **(a)** DSA, aortic arch injection performed via a pigtail catheter, showing a patent right brachiocephalic artery. Robust opacification of the right vertebral artery is now observed (*arrows*). **(b)** Fluoroscopy showing patent stent within the right brachiocephalic artery.

5 Internal Carotid Artery Occlusion

General Description

Clinical presentation of an isolated acute cervical internal carotid artery (ICA) occlusion can be quite variable, ranging from minimal, often fluctuating in severity, to profound neurologic deficits. Such variations in symptoms can be due to several factors, such as the degree of ICA occlusion (complete vs. severe flow-limiting stenosis), robustness of collaterals (circle of Willis and leptomeningeal collaterals), and the patient's hemodynamic and cardiac status. Acute ICA occlusion can be treated with balloon angioplasty alone or by placing a carotid stent. There is a risk of distal embolization into the anterior cerebral artery (ACA) and middle cerebral artery (MCA) territories; thus, an adequate embolic protection strategy, whether by a distal filter, proximal balloon, or both, is paramount.

Keywords: angioplasty, internal carotid artery, stenting

5.1 Anatomical and Imaging Aspects

- Magnetic resonance or computed tomography angiography (CTA) may not reliably distinguish true cervical occlusion from pseudo-occlusion or more distal occlusion compared with catheter angiography (▶ Fig. 5.1).

- A Mo.Ma proximal cerebral protection device (Medtronic) provides total flow arrest by occluding both the external carotid artery (ECA) and the common carotid artery (CCA), whereas balloon guide catheters (BGCs) only occlude the CCA. However, BGCs are more versatile from an anatomical perspective due to their higher trackability profile.

- The choice of endovascular devices depends on the anatomy and nature of the lesion (its length), degree of calcifications (▶ Fig. 5.2) and plaque ulcerations, presence of intraluminal clot (▶ Fig. 5.3), tortuosity of the cervical ICA, and risks associated with the use of antiplatelet agents in the acute setting (such as the use of glycoprotein IIb/IIIa inhibitors or single or dual-antiplatelet therapy, which may be required if a carotid stent is used) (▶ Fig. 5.1, ▶ Fig. 5.4).

5.2 Carotid Stent Selection

- Several stent options are available for the treatment of carotid origin stenosis or occlusion, many of which utilize the rapid-exchange design. Closed-cell, laser-cut stents (such as Xact

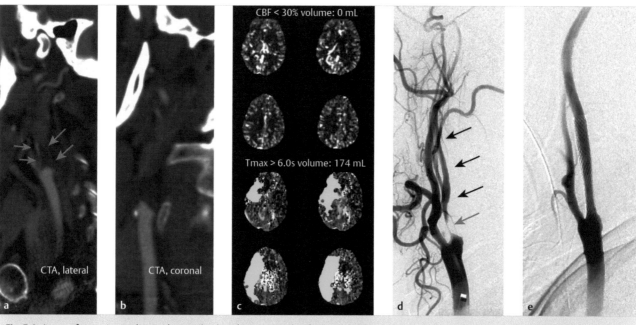

Fig. 5.1 A case of acute internal carotid artery (ICA) occlusion treated with stenting. **(a)** Computed tomography angiography (CTA) of the neck, lateral view, showing occluded origin of the right ICA. Hypodense "fresh" plaque is suspected (*arrows*). **(b)** CTA of the neck, coronal view. **(c)** Perfusion imaging shows a large perfusion deficit in the corresponding vascular territory. There is no ischemic core (cerebral blood flow [CBF] > 30%, which is used to estimate the size of stroke core, is 0 mL). Thus, it is relatively safe to use an aggressive antiplatelet regimen if needed. **(d)** Because of concern for clot disruption with angioplasty, primary stenting is chosen instead. Note that catheter angiography clearly shows impaired but still preserved anterograde filling of contrast material (*black arrows*) beyond the site of ICA origin critical occlusion (*red arrow*). The angiogram allows better appreciation of the extent of the stenotic lesion, making the intervention less challenging than in cases of complete occlusion. **(e)** Final angiogram performed after stenting showing restored patency of the ICA origin.

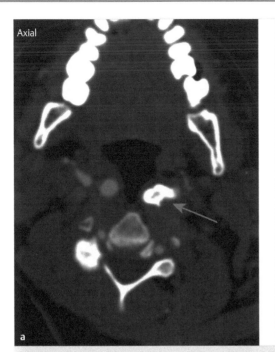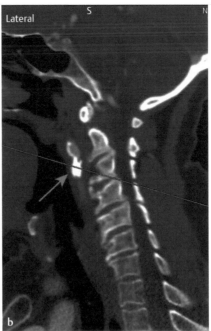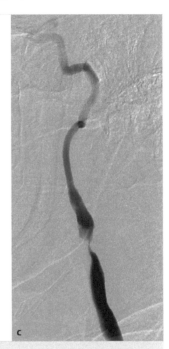

Fig. 5.2 Heavily calcified plaque with concentric calcification. **(a)** Axial computed tomography (CT) and **(b)** lateral CT showing extensive calcification (*red arrows*). A ring of heavily calcified plaque (concentric calcifications) will likely require a combination of angioplasty and stenting with a high radial force carotid stent to maintain patency of the internal carotid artery (ICA). **(c)** Digital subtraction angiography (DSA) shows critical stenosis of the ICA origin with faint filling of contrast beyond the occlusion.

[Abbott]) provide a high radial force that could make them ideal for cases with heavily calcified plaque (▶ Fig. 5.5). The downside of these stents is decreased ability to conform to a vessel wall, which is especially important in cases with tortuous anatomy.

- Braided stents (such as Wallstent [Boston Scientific]) provide additional coverage when oversized to the vessel diameter and may be beneficial in cases with long stenotic lesions.
- An open-cell design is more likely to cause plaque fragmentation during stenting (including poststenting balloon angioplasty).
- Selecting a short stent that only provides coverage of the stenotic area, especially in cases with major differences in ICA and CCA diameters, may result in immediate or delayed stent migration, the so-called "watermelon seeding" effect (▶ Fig. 5.6). Stent migration could be avoided by selecting a longer stent (in general, oversizing is less likely to create a problem than undersizing when it comes to selecting stents for treating carotid stenosis).

5.3 Technique and Key Steps

- Choice and type of guide sheath depends on the nature of the carotid lesion and the most appropriate treatment strategy (distal filter, proximal balloon, or both), tortuosity of the aortic arch and the carotid arteries, and additional treatment planned, such as thrombectomy of a tandem intracranial occlusion.
- Radial artery access can be used for a conventional guide catheter, such as a 0.070-inch Envoy (Codman Neuro) or a 0.071-inch Benchmark (Penumbra). However, if the use of BGCs or the Mo.Ma device is planned, femoral artery access should be utilized, because of the need to use an 8-French (F) or 9F sheath.
- Guide catheter balloons are prepared with a 50% contrast solution using a one- or three-way stopcock and a syringe. For cases of proximal protection using a BGC or the Mo.Ma device, systemic heparinization with a goal-activated coagulation time of 250 to 300 seconds may be required;

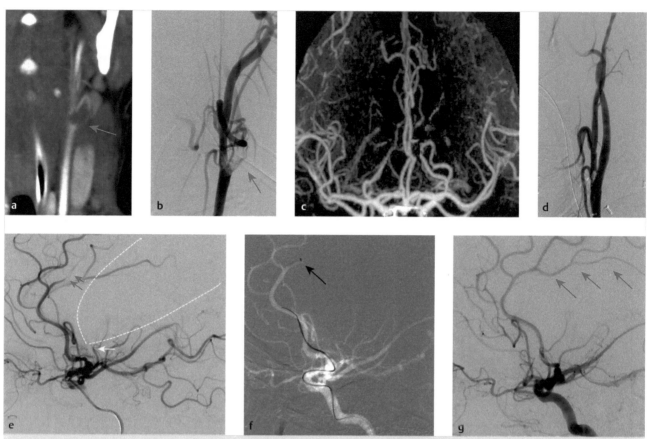

Fig. 5.3 An example of distal emboli released during carotid artery stenting in a case with underlying intraluminal thrombus. **(a)** Computed tomography angiography (CTA), anteroposterior (AP) view, showing a thrombus at the origin of the left internal carotid artery (ICA) (*red arrow*). **(b)** Digital subtraction angiography (DSA), AP view, confirms a fresh clot (*red arrow*). Extreme caution is needed to perform the intervention in this case, given the high risk for embolic complications. Lack of proper embolic protection when crossing the lesion and placing a stent may result in thrombus breakdown. **(c)** Downstream intracranial vessels prior to intervention are patent, as demonstrated by baseline intracranial CTA. **(d)** DSA, oblique view, demonstrating patent left ICA origin following placement of a stent. A long 6F sheath was used for access. **(e)** Upon performing an intracranial run, distal emboli in the anterior cerebral artery (ACA) (pericallosal branch, *red arrows*) are now noted (note that these branches were patent on the baseline CTA shown in c). There is also a major dropout of the left middle cerebral artery (MCA) from an M2 branch occlusion (*yellow arrow* points to the occlusion and the *dotted lines* indicate the corresponding affected downstream territory). The case needed to be converted to a thrombectomy intervention with thrombus aspiration and pharmacological thrombolysis with intra-arterial alteplase. **(f,g)** Lateral view, road map, and DSA, showing catheterization of the occluded anterior cerebral artery (ACA) branch with a 5F Sofia aspiration catheter (MicroVention) (*black arrow* in **f** points to the tip of the catheter) with a good angiographic outcome (*red arrows* in **g** correspond to the previously occluded distal ACA). Two 0.014-inch guidewires were used in this case for extra support in order to track the aspiration catheter around the ophthalmic segment and into the A1. Although adequate recanalization was eventually achieved, this rescue treatment could have been avoided with proper guide catheter selection (a balloon guide catheter would have been ideal in this case because the clot extended into both the ICA and ECA).

however, the extent of the infarct on baseline neuroimaging should be taken into account.

- A balloon insufflator is needed if angioplasty is planned. Similarly, a 50% contrast solution is adequate for balloon preparation. A percutaneous transluminal angioplasty balloon is chosen based on a measurement of the ICA beyond the lesion (when available). We prefer using an Aviator balloon (Cardinal Health). Occasionally, when stenosis is severe, a smaller profile predilatation balloon is needed.

- Aspiration through the guide catheter using 20-mL syringes will help remove the plaque debris trapped distal to the balloon. Aspirated samples can be filtered through a small particulate filter basket. One or two negative aspirates are needed before ensuring no residual debris is present before

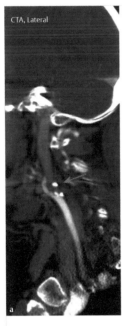

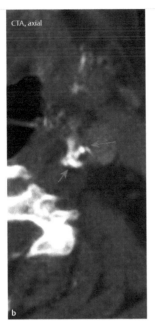

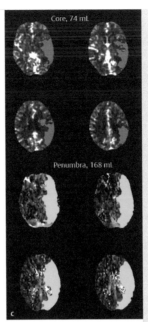

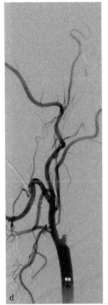

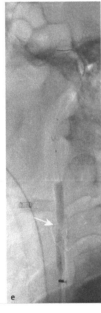

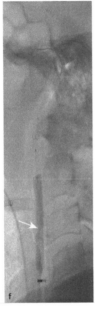

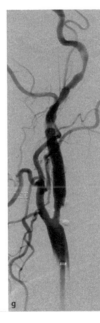

Fig. 5.4 An example of acute internal carotid artery (ICA) occlusion in a patient with a large ischemic core. **(a)** Computed tomography angiography (CTA), lateral view, shows complete occlusion of the left ICA origin (*arrow*). **(b)** CTA, axial view, showing "eccentric" scattered calcifications (*arrows*). **(c)** Computed tomography (CT) perfusion imaging shows a large ischemic core (measured by RAPID automated software [iSchemaView] at 74 mL). Emergent stenting would require the use of antiplatelet therapy, which in this case may increase the risk of reperfusion hemorrhage. **(d)** Digital subtraction angiography (DSA), lateral view, confirms complete occlusion of the ICA at its origin. **(e,f)** Angioplasty alone is performed. A series of rounds of angioplasty are needed before patency of the ICA is established (the *arrow* in each image points to the "waist" of the balloon, which corresponds to the maximal area of stenosis). A 5 × 40 mm Aviator balloon (Cardinal Health) is used here. **(g)** Postangioplasty injection shows approximately 50% residual stenosis of the ICA origin. Careful attention with repeat carotid ultrasound or CTA in 24 to 48 hours is needed to ensure that reocclusion does not develop. If follow-up head imaging shows no hemorrhagic transformation, definitive treatment of the lesion with carotid stenting or endarterectomy will likely be needed before the patient's discharge from the hospital.

deflating the balloon. In cases using a distal filter, filter aspiration can be performed using special aspiration catheters with rapid exchange capability, such as a 6F Export AP (Medtronic) or Pronto LP (Vascular Solutions).

- Intravascular ultrasound (IVUS; Volcano Corp.) can be used to evaluate for residual thrombus inside the stent.

5.4 Pearls and Pitfalls

- The guidewire should remain across the lesion until the procedure is complete. Acute reocclusion, repeat angioplasty, stent migration, or downstream occlusion may require additional treatment.

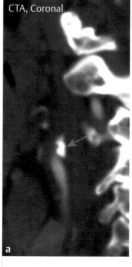 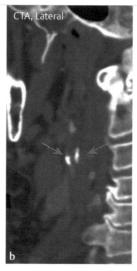 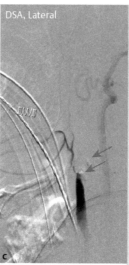

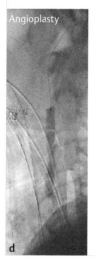 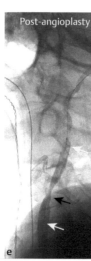 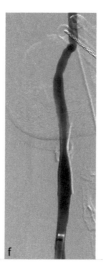 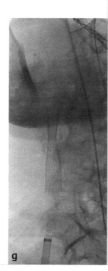

Fig. 5.5 Right internal carotid artery (ICA) occlusion with heavily calcified plaque. **(a)** Coronal and **(b)** lateral computed tomography angiography (CTA) views showing occlusion of the common carotid artery (CCA) bifurcation. Heavy calcifications at the origin of the right ICA are present (*arrows*). **(c)** Digital subtraction angiography (DSA), lateral views. Baseline run showing occlusion of the right ICA origin. Faint opacification of the ECA can be appreciated. Heavy calcified plaque is visualized on DSA (*arrows*). **(d)** Several rounds of angioplasty with an Aviator balloon fail to maintain adequate patency of the vessel and **(e)** postangioplasty (*black arrow* points to severe residual stenosis; *yellow arrows* indicate the balloon's markers); thus, emergent stenting is required. **(f)** DSA and **(g)** unsubstracted DSA views showing Xact stent (Abbott) deployed.

- Bradycardia and hypotension can occur during angioplasty. The anesthesia team should be alerted before performing angioplasty to have atropine or glycopyrrolate readily available. In cases of a significant blood pressure drop that is not responding to these anticholinergic agents, an infusion of dopamine may be required.
- Hyperperfusion can result in hemorrhagic transformation, especially in cases with a moderate or large size ischemic core. Aggressive blood pressure control maintained with systolic blood pressure in the 120–140 mmHg range may be needed immediately after the intervention.
- Patients treated with angioplasty alone should be closely monitored with repeat carotid ultrasound imaging or CTA in 24–72 hours. Reocclusion is not infrequent, and early definitive treatment with stenting or endarterectomy may be needed.

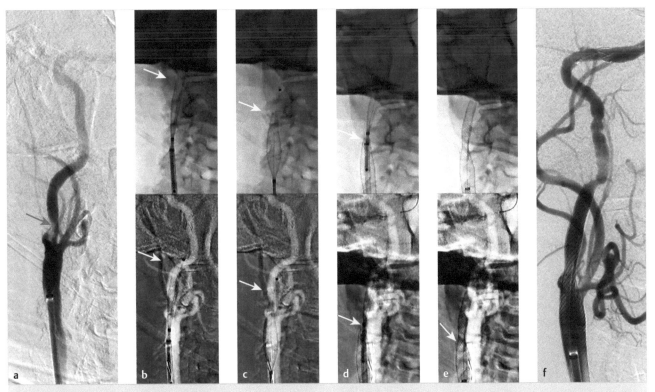

Fig. 5.6 An example of intraprocedural carotid stent migration requiring placement of a second stent. **(a)** Digital subtraction angiography (DSA), anteroposterior (AP) view, right common carotid artery (CCA) injection showing severe focal stenosis of the right internal carotid artery (ICA) origin (*arrow*). **(b)** Unsubtracted (top) and road map (bottom) views showing deployment of the stent (Wallstent [Boston Scientific]). The arrow in each image points to the distal end of the stent as it is being deployed. **(c)** Unsubtracted (top) and road map (bottom) views showing that downward migration of the stent into the CCA occurs during its deployment ("watermelon seeding"). The stenotic lesion is no longer covered by the stent (*arrow in each image*). Although the Wallstent could be resheathed during its partial deployment to adjust its landing zone, stent migration was recognized later in this case, i.e., after the stent was nearly fully deployed. **(d,e)** Unsubtracted (top) and road map (bottom) views. Placement of the second stent is now needed. The arrows correspond to the distal end of the first stent, showing its gradual downward migration. In **(e)**, the second stent is deployed. **(f)** Final angiographic run shows now patent right ICA.

5.5 Cases with Videos and Images

5.5.1 Case 5.1 Balloon Guide Catheter and Distal Filter for Cervical ICA Occlusion

In a patient with a fluctuating degree of left arm weakness, critical stenosis (often referred to as a pseudo-occlusion) of the right internal carotid artery (ICA) is discovered during the initial evaluation in the emergency department. Emergent stenting is planned. To minimize the risk of embolic complication, a combination of proximal (balloon guide catheter) and distal (embolic filter) embolic protection is chosen for the treatment strategy (▶ **Video 5.1**; ▶ Fig. 5.7, ▶ Fig. 5.8, ▶ Fig. 5.9, ▶ Fig. 5.10, ▶ Fig. 5.11, ▶ Fig. 5.12, ▶ Fig. 5.13).

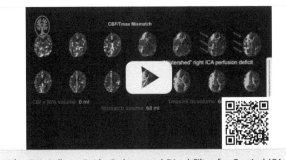

Video 5.1 Balloon Guide Catheter and Distal Filter for Cervical ICA Occlusion.

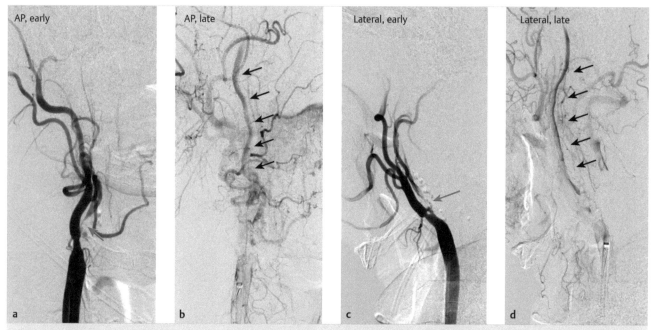

Fig. 5.7 Baseline angiography showing right internal carotid artery (ICA) occlusion. **(a,b)** Anteroposterior (AP) views, early and late arterial phase; and **(c,d)** lateral views, early and late arterial phase, of a right cervical angiogram. Highly calcified vulnerable plaque causing flow-limiting stenosis of the right ICA is shown at the arrow. Note the delayed filling of the ICA intracranially in the late arterial phase ("late") in comparison to the external carotid artery (ECA) branches robustly filling in the early arterial phase of the contrast injection ("early").

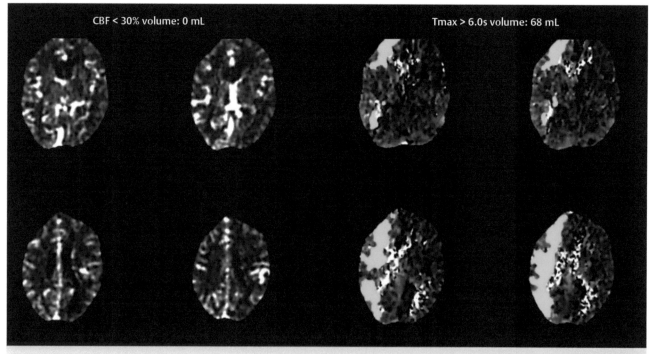

Fig. 5.8 Computed tomography (CT) perfusion. Perfusion maps show the right hemisphere at risk with a watershed perfusion defect, confirming the critical nature of the internal carotid artery (ICA) origin stenosis.

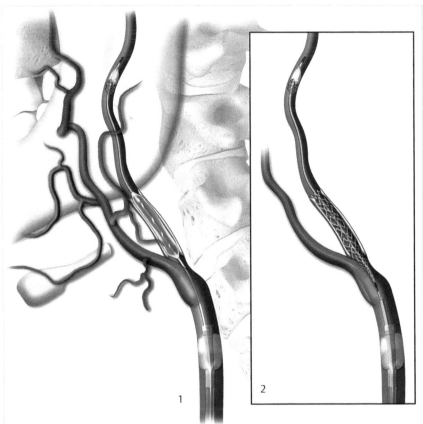

Fig. 5.9 Artist's illustration of the combined approach to embolic protection. Illustration demonstrates the combined approach of proximal protection using flow arrest with a BGC and distal filter ("belt and suspenders"). Following preangioplasty (step 1), stenting is performed (step 2). In case of critical stenosis as shown here, preangioplasty is required to cross the lesion for stent delivery and deployment. (© Thieme/ Jennifer Pryll)

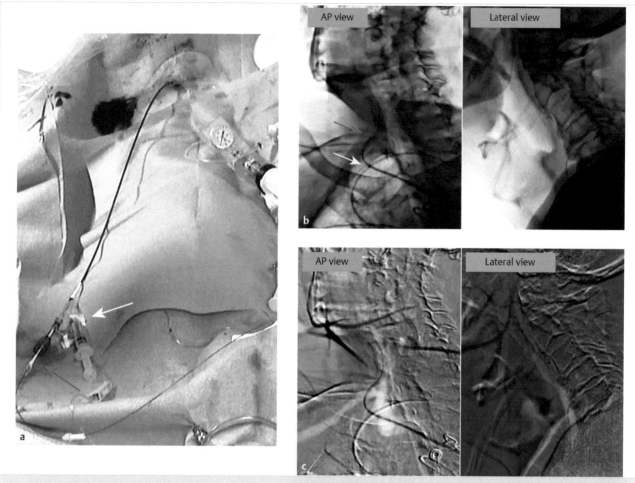

Fig. 5.10 Establishing access with a BGC. **(a)** After establishing groin access with a 9F sheath, a balloon guide catheter (BGC) is navigated into the distal common carotid artery (CCA) over a 0.035-inch guidewire and VTK catheter (Cook Medical; indicated with the *red arrow*). The BGC is prepped using a one-way stopcock and syringe filled with 50% contrast (*white arrow*). **(b)** Live fluoroscopy (anteroposterior [AP] and lateral views) and **(c)** roadmap (AP and lateral views) show careful navigation of the guidewire to avoid disturbing the plaque region. Once the wire is placed into the external carotid artery (ECA), the BGC (the *yellow arrow* points at the tip of BGC) can be delivered over the VTK (*red arrow*). In general, a 0.035-inch or a 0.038-inch guidewire is used depending on the arch anatomy. Most BGCs are quite rigid when compared with conventional guide catheters. An intermediate catheter such as a VTK is used to establish access. The balloon can be transiently inflated in the proximal CCA to facilitate delivery of the guide catheter in cases of tortuous anatomy,

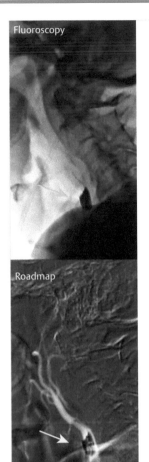
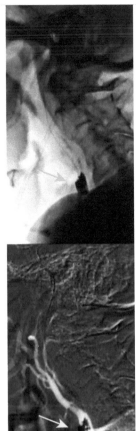
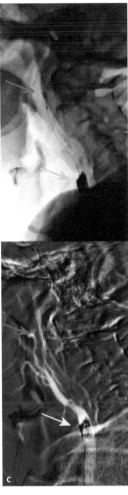

Fluoroscopy

Roadmap

a   b   c

Fig. 5.11 Distal filter placement. **(a–c)** Angiography, lateral view, live fluoroscopy images (top) and roadmap series (bottom), sequential images, showing carefully crossing the lesion with a 0.014-inch guidewire followed by distal filter placement at the C1 segment (*red arrow*). The BGC balloon at the CCA level is now fully inflated (*yellow arrow*) and will remain inflated until stenting is completed. Femoral artery access is used because an 8 or 9F sheath is required.

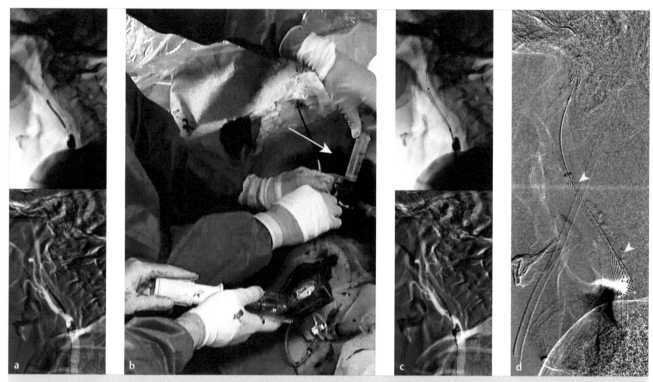

Fig. 5.12 Angioplasty and stenting. **(a)** Live procedural fluoroscopy images (top) and roadmap series (bottom) showing key procedural steps. Once balloon angioplasty is performed, aspiration through the guide catheter allows the removal of clot debris (top, live fluoroscopy images; bottom, roadmap series). Overinflation of the balloon of the balloon guide catheter (BGC) should be avoided. These balloons are easy to rupture. Also, when repositioning the guide catheter, the balloon must be at least partially deflated; otherwise, balloon rupture may occur. Gentle putting of contrast material through the guide catheter and its stasis or rapid washout can gauge whether the balloon is adequately inflated for optimal flow arrest during the intervention. **(b)** The photograph shows that one operator is deflating the angioplasty balloon while the second operator is aspirating through the guide catheter with a 20-mL syringe (*white arrow*). The angioplasty balloon is exchanged for a stent using the rapid exchange system. **(c)** The stent is deployed by pushing the device forward to maximize its radial force (top, live fluoroscopy images; bottom, roadmap series). **(d)** Final unsubtracted view shows fully deployed stent (*yellow arrowheads*). A Wallstent (Boston Scientific) was chosen for this case; this is a braided stent that performs favorably when there is a major discrepancy between the diameters of the internal carotid artery (ICA) and common carotid artery (CCA).

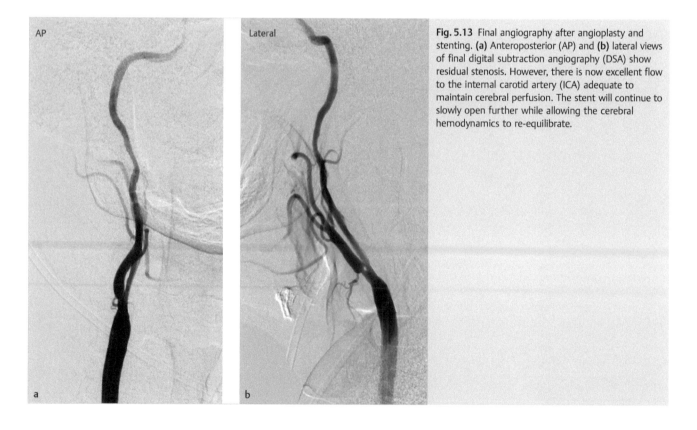

Fig. 5.13 Final angiography after angioplasty and stenting. **(a)** Anteroposterior (AP) and **(b)** lateral views of final digital subtraction angiography (DSA) show residual stenosis. However, there is now excellent flow to the internal carotid artery (ICA) adequate to maintain cerebral perfusion. The stent will continue to slowly open further while allowing the cerebral hemodynamics to re-equilibrate.

5.5.2 Case 5.2 Mo.Ma Device for ICA Occlusion

A patient is admitted to the emergency department with acute ischemic stroke. The examination is indicative of a right hemispheric syndrome, and neuroimaging shows near-occlusion of the right internal carotid artery (ICA) origin. Emergent stenting is planned, given the flow-limiting nature of the stenosis. There is evidence of a long ulcerated plaque lesion on neuroimaging; therefore, stenting with flow arrest using Mo.Ma device is planned (▶ **Video 5.2**; ▶ Fig. 5.14, ▶ Fig. 5.15, ▶ Fig. 5.16, ▶ Fig. 5.17, ▶ Fig. 5.18, ▶ Fig. 5.19, ▶ Fig. 5.20).

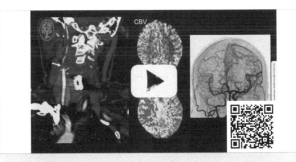

Video 5.2 Mo.Ma Device for ICA Occlusion.

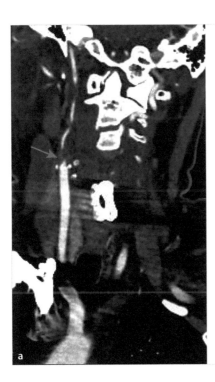
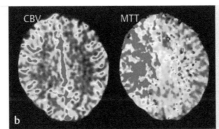
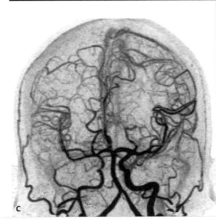

Fig. 5.14 Baseline imaging performed in the emergency department. **(a)** Computed tomography angiography (CTA) images demonstrating critical right internal carotid artery (ICA) origin occlusion (*arrow*) with a soft plaque as well as presence of calcifications. **(b)** Computed tomography (CT) perfusion maps show increased cerebral blood volume (CBV; left) and mean transit time (MTT; right) within the right middle cerebral artery (MCA) territory. **(c)** CTA reconstruction of intracranial vasculature shows an otherwise patent MCA. Such a significant hypoperfused state is due to the flow-limiting nature of the right ICA origin stenosis.

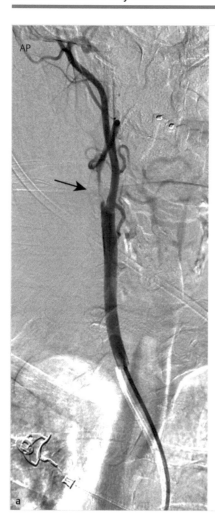 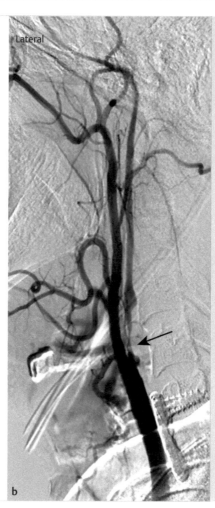

Fig. 5.15 Baseline angiography in the angiography suite. **(a)** Anteroposterior (AP) and **(b)** lateral views of baseline digital subtraction (DS) imaging runs showing near (pseudo) occlusion of the right internal carotid artery (ICA) origin (*arrow* in each image) with a very severe stenosis (>95%). Note faint and delayed filling of the ICA with contrast in comparison to the robust filling of the external carotid artery (ECA) branches. This indicates the hemodynamic nature of the stenosis. Given the evidence for a highly vulnerable plaque, proximal protection with the Mo.Ma device is chosen. A 9F sheath is required. Thus, femoral artery access is typically used.

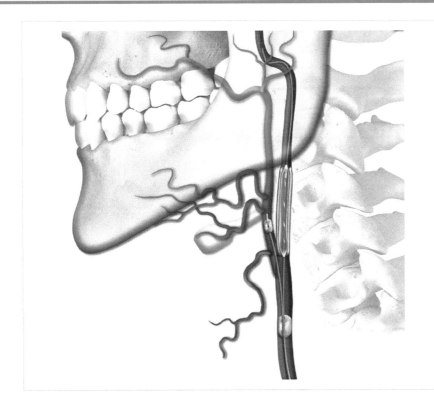

Fig. 5.16 Artist's illustration of the Mo.Ma device. The principle of complete flow arrest with the Mo.Ma device. Once both the external carotid artery (ECA) and common carotid artery (CCA) balloons are inflated, complete flow arrest with embolic protection is achieved. Radiopaque markers are centrally located in each balloon. Proximal (CCA) balloon occlusion range is 5–13 mm, distal (ECA) balloon occlusion range is 3–6 mm. A 0.014-inch guidewire is introduced across the lesion, allowing safe performance of balloon angioplasty. Debris is removed by blood aspiration. Mo.Ma is a double occlusion balloon system providing proximal embolic protection for carotid artery angioplasty and stenting. The inner diameter of the working channel is 2.12 mm (0.083 inch). Thus, the Mo.Ma device may not be ideal for use in cases of stroke with tandem intracranial occlusion when large bore intermediate catheter use is planned. (© Thieme/Jennifer Pryll)

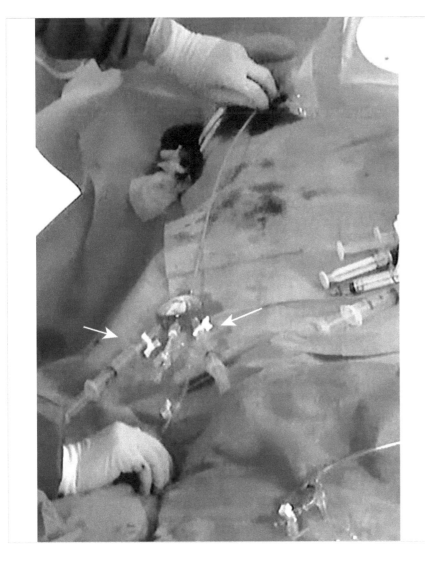

Fig. 5.17 Photograph demonstrating delivery of the Mo.Ma device via 9F sheath access. Once the guidewire is placed into the external carotid artery (ECA) using the exchange technique, the diagnostic catheter is removed and the device is delivered into the target region. The common carotid artery (CCA) and ECA balloons are already prepared using syringes filled with 50% contrast material and one-way stopcocks (*white arrows*).

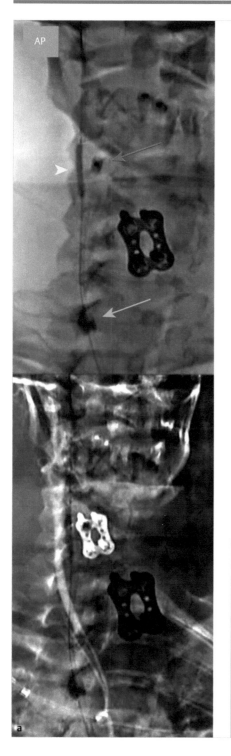
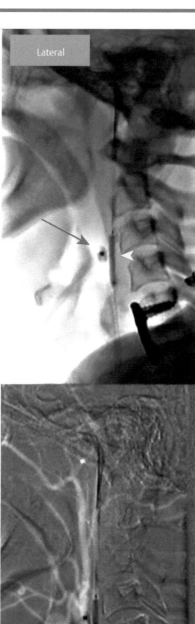

Fig. 5.18 Balloon angioplasty. **(a)** Anteroposterior (AP) and **(b)** lateral views, live fluoroscopy images (top), and roadmap series (bottom), of digital subtraction angiography (DSA) showing correct positioning of the Mo.Ma device. The external carotid artery (ECA) (*red arrow*) and common carotid artery (CCA) balloons (*green arrow*) are inflated before the lesion is crossed with a guidewire and angioplasty (*yellow arrowhead*) is performed. Both balloons remain inflated until stenting is performed.

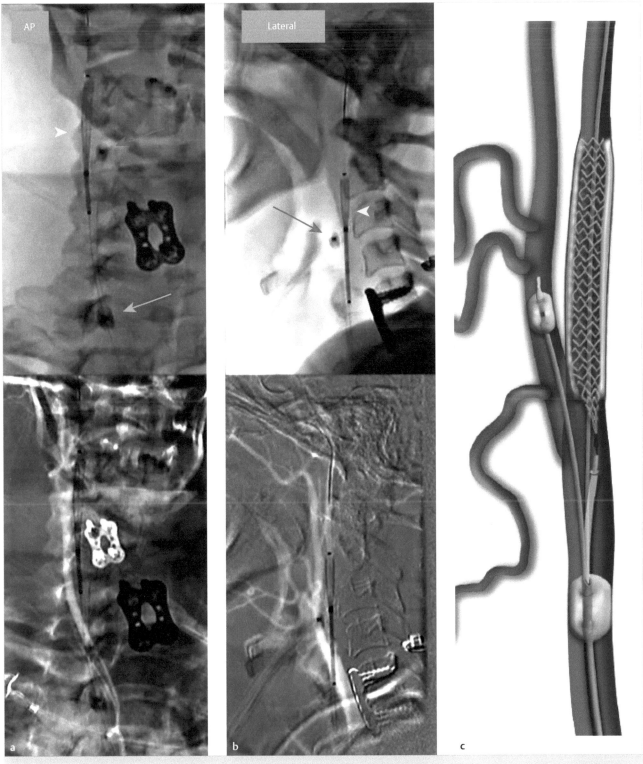

Fig. 5.19 Key steps of internal carotid artery (ICA) stenting. **(a)** Anteroposterior (AP) and **(b)** lateral views of digital subtraction angiography (DSA) (top, live fluoroscopy images; bottom, roadmap series), showing stent deployment (*yellow arrows*). The *red arrows* point at the external carotid artery (ECA) balloon, which is deflated first. After stent deployment is performed, aspiration from the guide catheter is performed prior to common carotid artery (CCA) balloon deflation (*green arrow*). **(c)** Artist's rendition of stent deployment during flow arrest (*purple color*) achieved by inflating ECA and CCA balloons. (**c:** © Thieme/Jennifer Pryll)

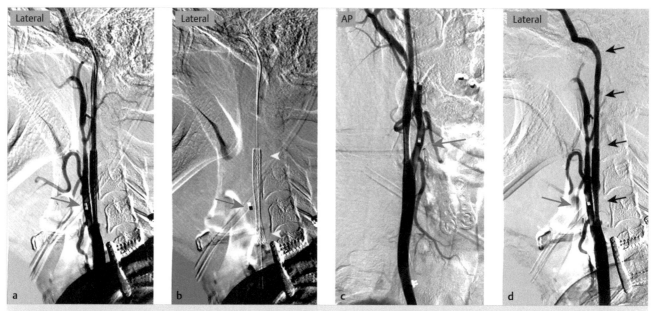

Fig. 5.20 Postintervention radiographic result. **(a–d)** Anteroposterior (AP) and lateral projections of final digital subtraction angiography (DSA) showing significant improvement in patency of the internal carotid artery (ICA) origin following stent placement (*yellow arrowheads*). The external carotid artery (ECA; *red arrow*) and common carotid artery (CCA) balloon (not shown) are now fully deflated.

5.5.3 Case 5.3 Unprotected Stenting and Distal Embolization

For this case of isolated acute right internal carotid artery (ICA) occlusion, radial artery access is chosen and stenting under distal embolic protection is planned. The case illustrates potential embolic complications that could occur during emergent angioplasty and stenting (▶ **Video 5.3**; ▶ Fig. 5.21, ▶ Fig. 5.22, ▶ Fig. 5.23, ▶ Fig. 5.24).

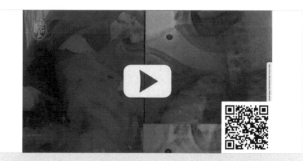

Video 5.3 Unprotected Stenting and Distal Embolization.

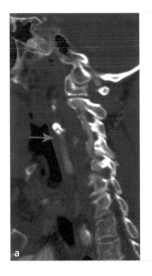

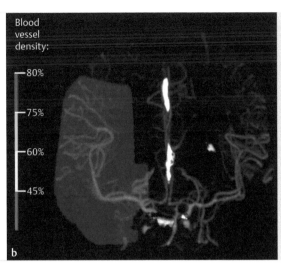

Blood
vessel
density:

—80%

—75%

—60%

—45%

Fig. 5.21 Initial imaging in the emergency department. **(a)** Computed tomography angiography (CTA), lateral view, demonstrating occlusion of the right internal carotid artery (ICA) origin (*red arrow*). A heavily calcified plaque is present at the C3 spinal level. **(b)** 3D reconstruction of the intracranial vasculature shows that the right middle cerebral artery (MCA) is in fact patent, with just minimally reduced vessel density. This indicates that the right hemisphere is perfused via the circle of Willis, confirming an isolated right ICA origin occlusion.

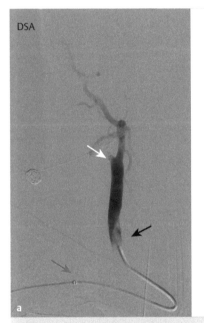

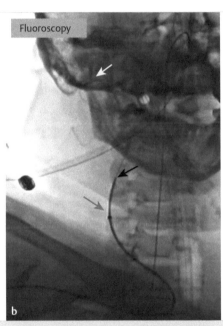

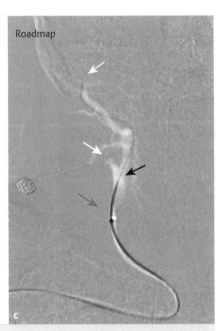

Fig. 5.22 Guide catheter access. **(a)** Digital subtraction angiography (DSA). **(b)** Live fluoroscopy, and **(c)** roadmap working projections showing steps to obtaining guide catheter access to the right common carotid artery (CCA). A Benchmark 071 guide catheter (Penumbra) was chosen (*red arrow*). A 5F Simmons 2 catheter (Merit Medical) is used for navigation (*black arrow*). Note how the 0.0035-inch guidewire (*yellow arrow*) is placed into the external carotid artery (ECA) to avoid contact with the occlusion site (*white arrow*). No balloon guide catheter (BGC) or distal embolic protection is used.

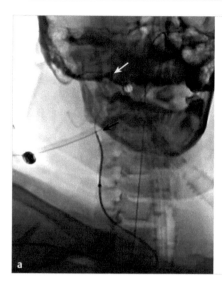
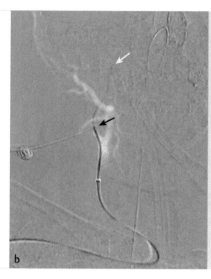

Fig. 5.23 Crossing the lesion. **(a)** Live fluoroscopy and **(b)** roadmap cervical views. Despite multiple attempts to cross the lesion with a 0.014-inch guidewire, all attempts were unsuccessful; and thus, a distal filter could not be advanced beyond the occlusion site. Thus, the 0.0035-inch guidewire (*yellow arrow*) and Simmons 2 catheter (*black arrow*) were used to cross this heavily calcified occlusion.

Angioplasty

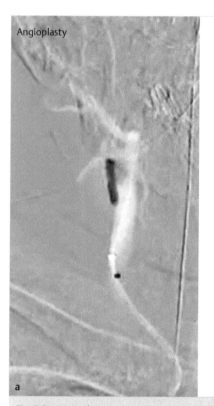

Stenting

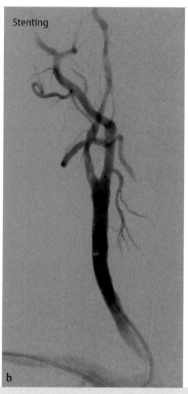

Distal emboli

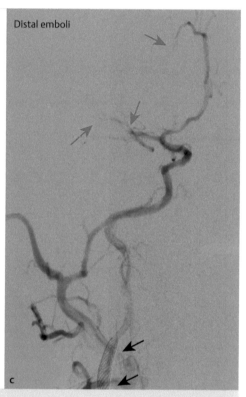

Fig. 5.24 Angioplasty and stenting. **(a)** Live fluoroscopy and **(b)** angiography. Following balloon angioplasty and stenting, patency of the right internal carotid artery (ICA) origin was established. **(c)** Angiogram after stenting shows extensive distal embolization (*red arrows*). *Black arrows* are pointing at the fresh carotid stent (Wallstent). This case required conversion to middle cerebral artery (MCA) thrombectomy to treat this new occlusion, which was likely the result of unprotected ICA angioplasty and stenting. Proximal or distal protection is paramount for such cases to avoid distal embolization complications.

6 Internal Carotid Artery Dissection

General Description

Acute carotid artery dissection causing acute ischemic stroke warrants emergent endovascular intervention if the dissection results in flow-limiting stenosis or causes complete internal carotid artery (ICA) occlusion. In those cases in which a tandem downstream occlusion is present, even a non-flow-limiting dissection may require emergent stenting to establish distal access with a guide catheter. The etiology is often traumatic or iatrogenic, although it is not uncommon to encounter patients with spontaneous dissection in the emergency department presenting with stroke symptoms. Dissection is a common cause of stroke in young patients. Anticoagulation or antiplatelet therapy is reserved for patients presenting with a stable neurological examination or minimal symptoms not warranting intervention. Stenting is highly effective in treating this specific vascular etiology of stroke.

Keywords: carotid dissection, carotid stent, intracranial stent

6.1 Anatomical and Imaging Aspects

- The dissection often begins distal to the takeoff of the ICA and can extend into the petrous segment or even intracranially.
- Computed tomography angiography (CTA) and magnetic resonance angiography (MRA) may demonstrate vessel wall irregularities, gradual tapering of the vessel (best seen with catheter angiography; the so-called "flame sign"), an intimal flap, and adjacent thrombus (▶ Fig. 6.1, ▶ Fig. 6.2). The mechanism of stroke can be embolic, hemodynamic (first affecting "watershed" territories; ▶ Fig. 6.1), or both.
- Pseudoaneurysm formation can occur, creating a reservoir for clot formation as a source of potential stroke in the future.

6.2 Carotid Stent Selection

- The goal of endovascular treatment is to restore cerebral blood flow. There is no need for extraradial force to normalize the vessel caliber; the choice of stent largely depends on the extent of the lesion (cervical only or involving petrous and/or cavernous segments), vessel diameter, and tortuosity.
- Open-cell laser-cut carotid stents (Acculink [Abbott Vascular]), a braided carotid stent design (Wallstent [Boston Scientific]), traditional intracranial stents (Atlas [Stryker], Enterprise [Johnson & Johnson], Wingspan [Stryker]), or even stents with flow diverter properties (Surpass [Stryker], Pipeline embolization device [Medtronic]) could all be used depending on the anatomical features of the lesion (▶ Fig. 6.3).
- Covered stents should be avoided. Currently available covered stents are extremely rigid and likely to cause additional dissection when attempting to deliver the stent.

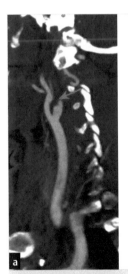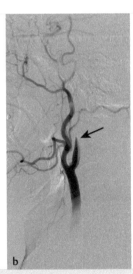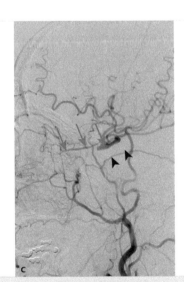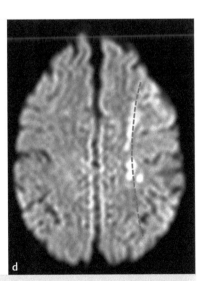

Fig. 6.1 Cervical internal carotid artery (ICA) dissection as a cause of watershed stroke. **(a)** Computed tomography angiography (CTA) and **(b)** digital subtraction angiography (DSA), lateral views, showing a typical flame-shaped cutoff of the cervical ICA (*arrow* in each image). This filling defect often begins at or just distal to the carotid bifurcation and slowly tapers more distally. **(c)** DSA, lateral view, intracranial projection, showing reconstitution of the ICA intracranially (*arrowheads*) via the ophthalmic artery (*arrows*) through anastomoses with the external carotid artery branches. **(d)** Magnetic resonance angiography (MRA) showing acute infarction in the distribution of anterior cerebral artery and middle cerebral artery (MCA) watershed territories (*broken line*), as a result of hypoperfusion caused by the ICA dissection.

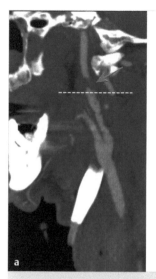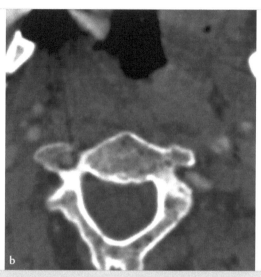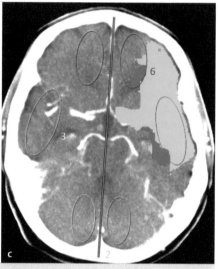

Fig. 6.2 Distal cervical internal carotid artery (ICA) dissection. **(a)** Lateral and **(b)** axial computed tomography angiography (CTA) views showing near occlusion of the distal cervical ICA caused by a dissection. Note that the dissection starts rather proximally, essentially at the carotid bifurcation, but the flow-limiting stenosis is present only distally (as seen by the vessel dropout indicated with the *arrow* in **(a)**. The *broken line* in **(a)** shows the level of the axial projection. **(c)** Computed tomography (CT) perfusion image showing a corresponding perfusion deficit in the downstream middle cerebral artery (MCA) territory. There is a large area of hypoperfused tissue at risk (*green color* represents ischemic "penumbra") for permanent ischemic damage if emergent revascularization is not performed.

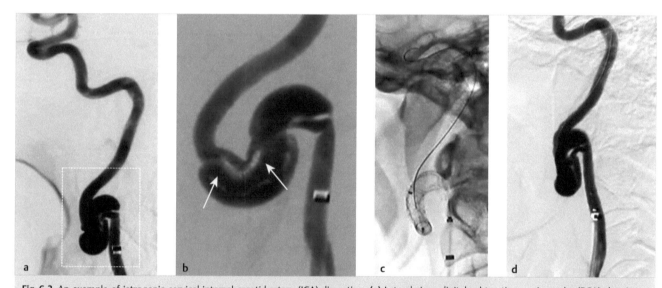

Fig. 6.3 An example of iatrogenic cervical internal carotid artery (ICA) dissection. **(a)** Lateral view, digital subtraction angiography (DSA) showing severe tortuosity of the cervical ICA segment. This patient had a recent endovascular intervention and a dissection was caused while placing a guide catheter. Such vascular injury could be avoided by using soft navigable intermediate catheters while parking the guide sheath proximal to such a high-risk anatomical area. The area within the broken rectangle is magnified in panel **b**. **(b)** DSA, high magnification image showing that treatment of the dissection was initially attempted by placing an intracranial stent (low-profile visualized intramural support [LVIS; MicroVention], shown by the *arrows*). Because that stent was too short and small in diameter in comparison to the size of the vessel, this maneuver was not successful. **(c)** Live fluoroscopy image showing a repeat procedure performed, this time using a different stent type (Surpass [Stryker]). The Surpass stent is a more appropriate choice here, given its large dimensions and higher radial force in comparison to that of the LVIS. It also offers a robust flow diversion effect. **(d)** DSA, postprocedural view, lateral projection. The guidewire remains across the lesion until patency of the dissected segment is confirmed angiographically.

Table 6.1 Use of antiplatelet agents for emergent stenting

Agent	Time-to-peak effect	Duration of effect	Dosage	Elimination
Aspirin	1–2 h	7–10 d	325- to 650-mg loading dose, 81- to 325-mg maintenance	Renal
Clopldogrel	2–6 h	5–7 d	300- to 600-mg loading dose, 75-mg maintenance	Renal and gastrointestinal
Prasugrel (Effient [Eli Lilly and Company])	0.5–4 h	5–9 d	60-mg loading dose, 10-mg maintenance	Renal and gastrointestinal
Ticagrelor (Brilinta [AstraZeneca])	0.5–2 h	3–5 d	180-mg loading dose, 90-mg twice daily maintenance	Renal and gastrointestinal
Cangrelor	2–30 min	0–30 min	30 mcg/kg IV bolus, 4 mcg/kg/min IV infusion	Renal and gastrointestinal

Table 6.2 Use of glycoprotein IIb/IIIa inhibitors for emergent stenting

Agent	Bolus dose	Infusion dose	Half-life
Abciximab (ReoPro [Janssen Pharmaceuticals])	0.125 mg/kg	Not needed	10–30 min with antiplatelet effect lasting up to 48 h
Eptifibatide (Integrilin [Merck Sharp & Dohme])	180 μg/kg	0.5 μg/kg/min	2.5 h
Tirofiban (Aggrastat [Medicure])	0.4 μg/kg/min or none	0.1 μg/kg/min	2 h

- A loading dose of antiplatelet agents should be administered to the patient before the procedure if stenting of a dissection is planned (▶ Table 6.1). For those cases in which dissection is recognized in the angiography suite, intravenous administration of glycoprotein IIb/IIIa inhibitors is required before transitioning to oral agents (▶ Table 6.2).

6.3 Technique and Key Steps

- Placing a stent in a false dissection lumen is the most feared technical complication (▶ Fig. 6.4). Once this occurs, it is extremely challenging to catheterize the true lumen and such a mistake will likely cause complete vessel occlusion. To avoid this, the correct position in the true lumen can be carefully confirmed with a microcatheter injection of contrast material beyond the site of occlusion. Once the position of the true lumen has been confirmed by catheter angiography, a 0.014-inch exchange length guidewire is delivered into the microcatheter, and the exchange technique is used for stent delivery.
- The guidewire should remain across the lesion until patency of the entire vessel is confirmed by angiography. A common mistake is to cover the dissected segment only in part, leaving a portion of the dissection flap unsecured. The dissection often starts more proximally and ends more distally than the borders appreciated angiographically.
- If the dissection segment extends beyond the cervical ICA segment, devices with different properties may be needed (such as a carotid stent placed more proximally and a self-expandable laser-cut or braided intracranial stent positioned more distally).
- The arterial access approach (radial vs. femoral) and guide catheter choice will depend on the extent and nature of the dissecting lesion. In cases suspicious for the presence of intraluminal thrombus, the use of a balloon-guide catheter (BGC) or the Mo.Ma device (Medtronic) may be warranted to minimize the risk of distal embolic complications.

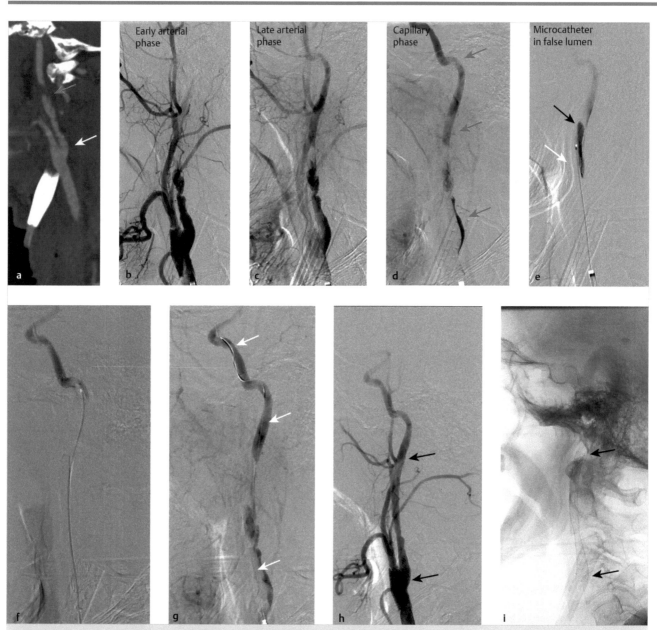

Fig. 6.4 Recognizing a true versus a false lumen when stenting a carotid dissection. **(a)** Computed tomography angiography (CTA) showing an extensive dissection starting at the carotid bifurcation (*white arrow*) and extending distally, where a near occlusion can be recognized (*red arrow*). **(b–d)** Digital subtraction angiography (DSA), lateral views of sequential arterial phases, showing the flow-limiting nature of the dissection. Note delated filling and stasis of contrast material (*arrows*) within the internal carotid artery (ICA) distal to the occlusion site. **(e)** DSA, lateral view, microcatheter injection shows that the tip of the microcatheter is within the false lumen of the dissection. Stenting this segment would result in complete occlusion of the vessel and thus should be carefully avoided. The *white arrows* correspond to the tip of the microcatheter. The *black arrow* indicates the false lumen of the dissection. **(f)** DSA, microcatheter injection confirms that the microcatheter is now positioned within the true lumen, as indicated by the flow of contrast material intracranially without opacification of the dissection lumen. **(g)** Once positioning of the microcatheter within the true vessel lumen is confirmed angiographically, an exchange length guidewire (*arrow*) can be used to remove the microcatheter for stent delivery. **(h)** DSA, lateral view, final run showing successful stenting of the dissected segment resulting in excellent vessel reconstruction. Note how a rather long stent (Wallsent, Boston Scientific) was chosen to ensure that the entire dissected segment of the ICA is adequately covered by the stent (*arrows*). **(i)** Fluoroscopy showing the location of the stent (*arrows*).

- Selecting a guide catheter with a large inner diameter (such as 6F) allows the use of a variety of stents. Oversized stents are preferable; stent design should be considered when selecting the most appropriate size (▶ Table 6.3). For instance, once unsheathed, braided stents will foreshorten if undersized, whereas significant oversizing will increase the length of vessel coverage.

6.4 Pearls and Pitfalls

- A dissected segment often begins more proximally and ends more distally than the area of dissection that is visualized angiographically. Unless there is a strong reason not to do so, when selecting a stent construct, covering a larger area will ensure that the entire diseased segment is adequately covered.
- The underlying etiology of dissection is vascular injury, and atherosclerosis or calcifications are rarely present. As such, selecting devices with the most radial force is rarely needed. Instead, the use of stents that are more likely to conform to the tortuous anatomy, such as braded or open-cell laser-cut stents, is preferable. Pre- or postdilatation is rarely needed unless there is concurrent underlying atherosclerotic disease.

Table 6.3 Carotid stent design

Stent	Design
Precise (Cardinal Health)	Open-cell
Protégé (Medtronic)	Open-cell, tapered
Wallstent (Boston Scientific)	Braided
Acculink (Abbott)	Open-cell
Xact (Abbott)	Closed-cell, tapered
Casper (MicroVention-Terumo)	Dual-layer design, braided

- Extreme caution is advised to avoid stenting the false lumen. Correction of such a technical complication is very challenging.

6.5 Cases with Videos and Images

6.5.1 Case 6.1 Stenting of Cervical Internal Carotid Artery (ICA) Dissection Under Flow Arrest

A young patient with a history of a motor vehicle accident several days earlier presents with left hemiparesis. A long segment of right internal carotid artery (ICA) dissection is recognized on an emergent computed tomography angiogram (CTA) of the head and neck. Stenting is planned under flow arrest using the Mo.Ma device (Medtronic) because of concern for a possible intraluminal thrombus and risk of embolic complications (▶ **Video 6.1**; ▶ Fig. 6.5, ▶ Fig. 6.6, ▶ Fig. 6.7, ▶ Fig. 6.8, ▶ Fig. 6.9, ▶ Fig. 6.10, ▶ Fig. 6.11).

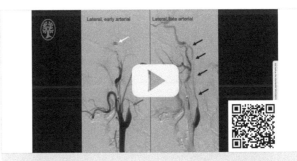

Video 6.1 Stenting of Cervical Internal Carotid Artery (ICA) Dissection Under Flow Arrest.

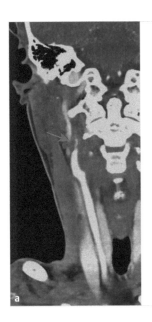

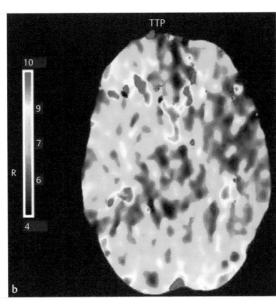

Fig. 6.5 Baseline noninvasive imaging. **(a)** Computed tomography angiography (CTA), coronal view, showing tapering of the right internal carotid artery (ICA). This is a common finding in carotid dissection, in contrast to an abrupt cutoff of the ICA origin seen in occlusions caused by atherosclerosis. **(b)** Computed tomography (CT) perfusion image showing increased time-to-peak (TTP) in the corresponding territory.

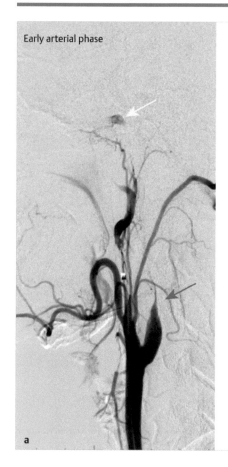

Early arterial phase

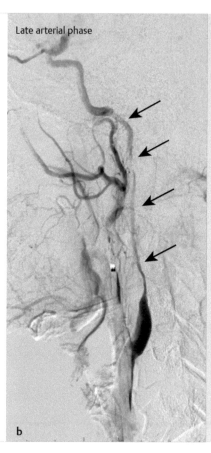

Late arterial phase

a

b

Fig. 6.6 Internal carotid artery (ICA) dissection is confirmed on catheter angiography. **(a)** Digital subtraction angiogram (DSA), lateral view, early arterial phase showing a flame-shaped occlusion (*red arrow*). The ICA fills distally via its petrous segment collaterals with the external carotid artery (ECA) first (*yellow arrow*). **(b)** DSA, later arterial phase with significantly delayed anterograde filling of the ICA (*arrows*).

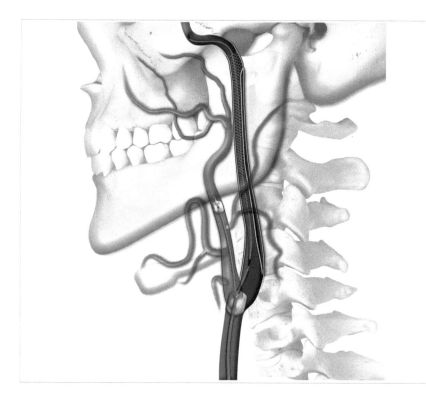

Fig. 6.7 Artist's illustration shows the plan to arrest flow in the external carotid artery (ECA) and common carotid artery (CCA) prior to stenting. (© Thieme/Jennifer Pryll)

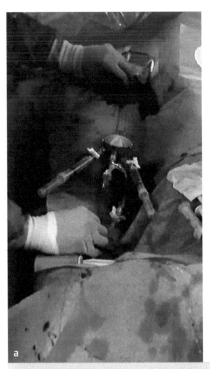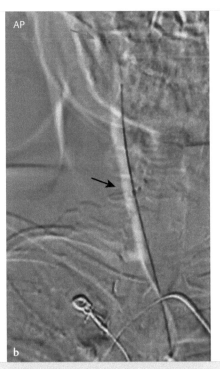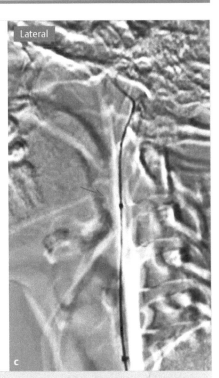

Fig. 6.8 Establishing access with Mo.Ma. **(a)** After placing a 9-French (F) sheath, a diagnostic catheter is used to deliver a guide catheter into the external carotid artery (ECA) and then exchanged for the Mo.Ma device. **(b)** Anteroposterior (AP) and **(c)** lateral views of intraprocedural digital subtraction angiography (DSA) roadmaps showing the Mo.Ma's distal balloon in the ECA (*red arrow*) and proximal balloon in the common carotid artery (CCA) (*black arrow*). The balloons have been prepared with 50% contrast material but not yet inflated.

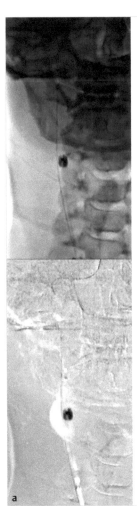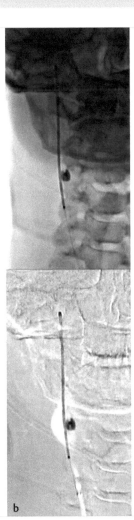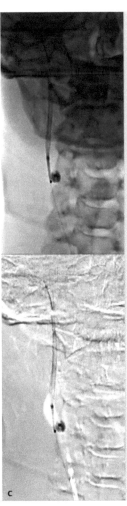

Fig. 6.9 Delivery and deployment of carotid stent. **(a–c)** Anteroposterior (AP) views, live fluoroscopy (top images) with corresponding roadmaps (bottom images), showing delivery and gradual deployment of Wallstent (Boston Scientific) under flow arrest. No angioplasty is needed. Choosing a large device (such as the 8 mm × 38 mm stent in this case) ensured that the entire diseased segment of the internal carotid artery (ICA) is adequately covered by the stent. Note that both balloons are fully inflated during this critical step. A change in balloon shape from cylindrical to circular may indicate the need for additional balloon inflation.

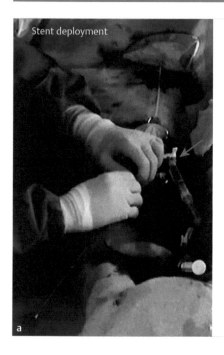

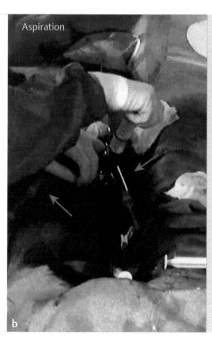

Fig. 6.10 Photographs of stent deployment. **(a)** Both external carotid artery (ECA) and common carotid artery (CCA) balloons remain inflated (*arrow*) during stent deployment. **(b)** Following stent deployment, blood is aspirated to remove clot debris before the Mo.Ma's balloons are deflated (*arrows*).

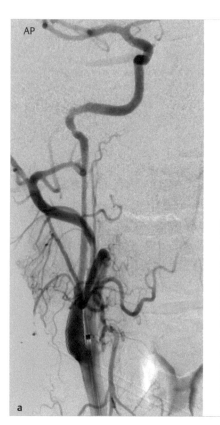

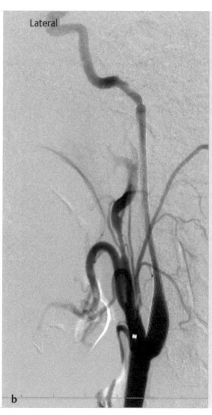

Fig. 6.11 Final angiographic result. **(a)** Antero-posterior (AP) and **(b)** lateral digital subtraction angiography (DSA) views, final postintervention common carotid artery (CCA) injection. With a single device, patency of the right internal carotid artery (ICA) is now established.

6.5.2 Case 6.2 Repair of a Long Dissection with Two Stents

In this case, a left internal carotid artery (ICA) dissection diagnosed during evaluation for acute ischemic stroke with left hemispheric syndrome was a surprising finding. There was no clear history of trauma, although the patient's family acknowledged recent seasonal allergies with frequent sneezing (▶ **Video 6.2**; ▶ Fig. 6.12, ▶ Fig. 6.13, ▶ Fig. 6.14, ▶ Fig. 6.15, ▶ Fig. 6.16, ▶ Fig. 6.17, ▶ Fig. 6.18).

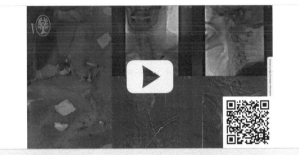

Video 6.2 Repair of a Long Dissection with Two Stents.

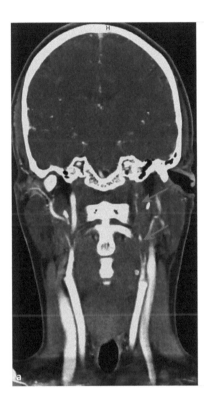

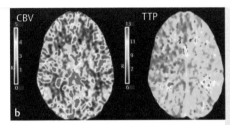

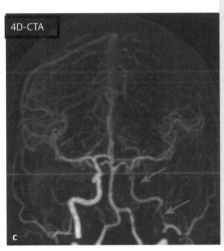

Fig. 6.12 Baseline noninvasive imaging suggestive of left internal carotid artery (ICA) occlusion. **(a)** Computed tomography angiography (CTA) showing dropout of the left ICA throughout its cervical, petrous, and more distal segments. A trickle of contrast flow is seen (*arrows*). **(b)** Perfusion maps show preserved cerebral blood volume (CBV) but impaired time-to-peak (TTP) of the left hemisphere. **(c)** Four-dimensional (4D) CTA, also known as "dynamic" CTA, demonstrates diminished filling of the left ICA (*arrows*).

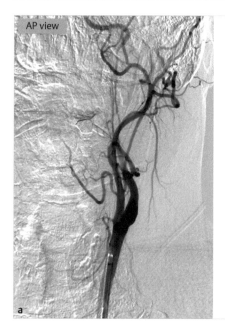

AP view

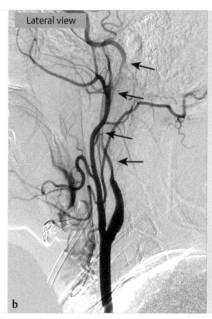

Lateral view

Fig. 6.13 Baseline angiography confirming left internal carotid artery (ICA) dissection. **(a)** Anteroposterior (AP) and **(b)** lateral digital subtraction angiography (DSA) views showing the extent of the dissection including the petrous segment of the left ICA (*arrows*).

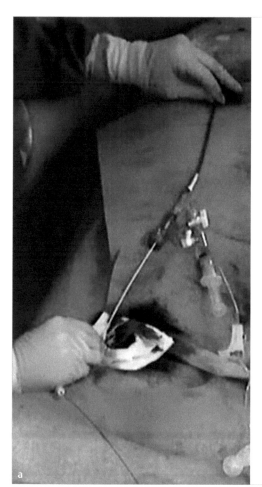

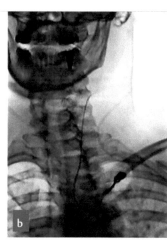

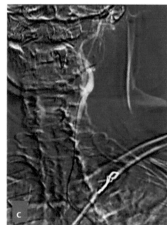

Fig. 6.14 Internal carotid artery (ICA) access with a guide catheter. **(a)** Stenting using flow arrest with a balloon guide catheter (BGC) is chosen as the treatment strategy. The BGC is delivered with the assistance of a VTK intermediate catheter (Cook Medical) and a 0.035-inch guidewire. **(b)** Live fluoroscopy (top image) and **(c)** roadmap (bottom image), digital subtraction angiography (DSA), anteroposterior (AP) view, showing delivery of the BGC.

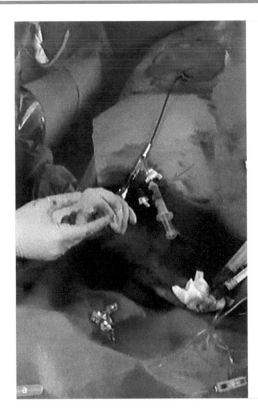

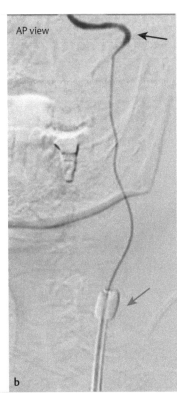

Fig. 6.15 Balloon inflation. (a) Photograph and (b) digital subtraction angiography (DSA) showing that once the balloon guide catheter (BGC) is in place, the balloon is inflated (*red arrows*) and a gentle injection of contrast material through the microcatheter is performed to confirm that the dissected segment is fully crossed and the microcatheter is positioned in the vessel's true lumen (*black arrow*).

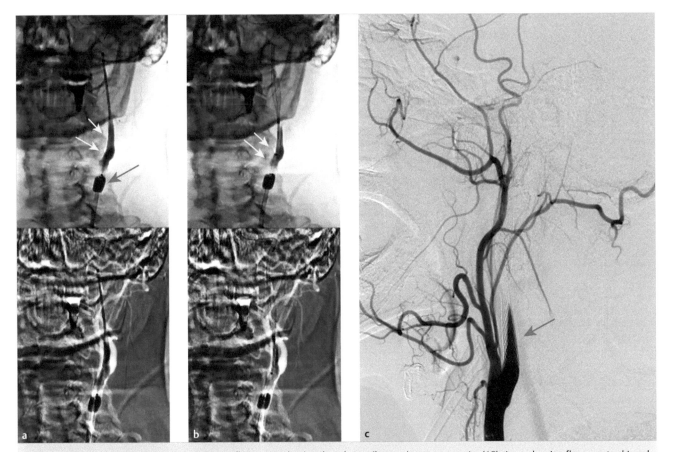

Fig. 6.16 Stent deliver and deployment. (a,b) Live fluoroscopy (top) and roadmaps (bottom), anteroposterior (AP) views, showing flow arrest achieved by inflating the balloon. Note the cylindrical shape of the balloon (*red arrow*). Contrast stasis after a gentle contrast puff confirms complete flow arrest achieved in this case (*yellow arrows*) as the stent (Wallstent) is positioned in place and unsheathed. (c) However, following stent deployment, the digital subtraction angiography (DSA) shows lack of robust contrast opacification (*arrow*) indicating downstream occlusion. The likely explanation for this angiographic finding is further extension of the dissection beyond the distal end of the stent, requiring additional stent placement.

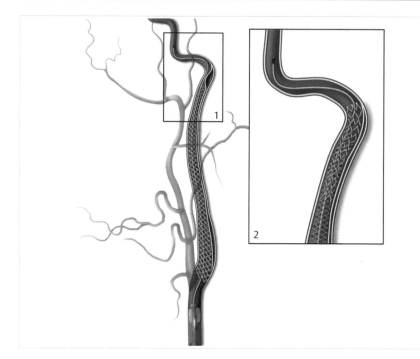

Fig. 6.17 Artist's illustration showing suboptimal result after first stent placement. A persistent flow-limiting dissection just distal to the first placed stent (1), explaining how a second stent is needed to repair this segment in order to restore flow through the entire internal carotid artery (ICA) (2). (© Thieme/Jennifer Pryll)

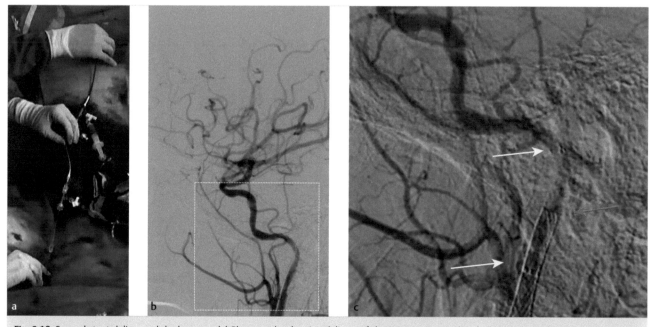

Fig. 6.18 Second stent deliver and deployment. **(a)** Photography showing delivery of the Wingspan stent (Stryker). This is a self-expanding, laser-cut, nitinol stent. Examples of other types of laser-cut stents that could be used here are Enterprise (Johnson & Johnson) or Atlas (Stryker). **(b)** Standard and **(c)** high-magnification lateral digital subtraction angiography (DSA) views showing that patency of the internal carotid artery (ICA) is now fully restored. The Wingspan stent (*yellow arrows*) is overlapping with the Wallstent (*red arrow*).

7 Internal Carotid Artery Terminus Occlusion

General Description

The term internal carotid artery (ICA) terminus (ICA-T) is used rather loosely in this chapter because the main principles of thrombectomy described here will also apply for cases with the embolus (thrombus) found at a more proximal location, such as the cavernous or paraclinoid segment of the ICA. ICA-T occlusions are often characterized by high clot burden and rapid infarct progression as a result of compromised collaterals within the circle of Willis. In this chapter, we review the nuances of aspiration, stent retriever (SR) thrombectomy, and intracranial angioplasty and/or stenting in this population of patients. The technique of aspiration and SR thrombectomy is reviewed in detail in the middle cerebral artery (MCA) chapters 9, 10 and 11 of this atlas.

Keywords: Balloon guide catheter, internal carotid artery terminus, stent retriever, stenting, thrombectomy

7.1 Anatomical and Imaging Aspects

- Determining the precise location of an ICA occlusion on noninvasive imaging can be challenging. On magnetic resonance angiography (MRA) and computed tomography angiography (CTA), the occlusion often appears to be located more proximally than its true level as a result of delayed filling of the ICA stump (▶ Fig. 7.1).
- On diagnostic subtraction angiography (DSA), selective ICA catheterization with the guide catheter and allowing additional time for the contrast material to reach the occlusion help determine the true extent of the occlusion. Opacification (or lack of it) of the ICA branches (such as the ophthalmic, posterior communicating, or anterior choroidal arteries) helps gauge the proximal end of the occlusive clot (▶ Fig. 7.2).

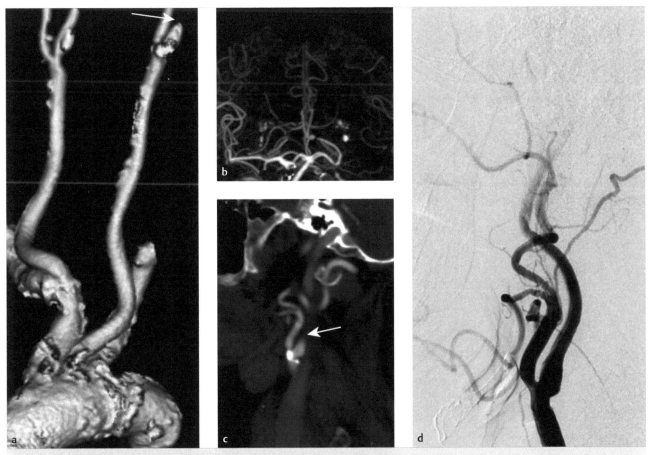

Fig. 7.1 Internal carotid artery (ICA) occlusion diagnosed with computed tomography angiography (CTA) and digital subtraction angiography (DSA). **(a)** Cervical CTA, three-dimensional (3D) reconstruction, showing occlusion of the left ICA just near its origin (*arrow*). **(b)** Cranial CTA, 3D reconstruction, demonstrating absence of the left ICA and middle cerebral artery (MCA). **(c)** CTA, lateral view, with gradual tapering of the left ICA just distal to the carotid bifurcation (*arrow*). **(d)** DSA, lateral view, left common carotid artery (CCA) injection. Unlike the previous image, here gradual filling of the entire cervical ICA with contrast material can be appreciated, but the precise level of ICA occlusion remains unclear.

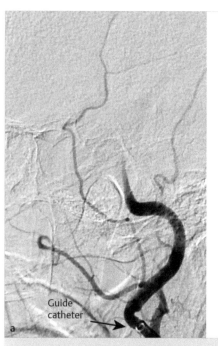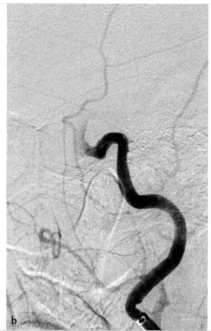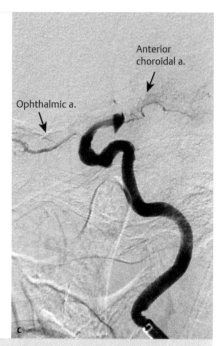

Fig. 7.2 Determining the exact location of internal carotid artery (ICA) occlusion on digital subtraction angiography (DSA). **(a–c)** DSA, lateral view, left ICA injection. Allowing extra time for contrast material to reach the occlusion eventually opacifies the ophthalmic and anterior choroidal arteries. More precise location of the proximal end of the clot can now be appreciated, aiding the interventionist with sizing and placement of the thrombectomy device. The guide catheter is seen in the cervical left ICA.

- In patients with poor collaterals, CTA or MRA may not display how far the clot extends. To ensure that an SR adequately captures the entire clot, a selective injection through a microcatheter is performed (▶ Fig. 7.3).
- A heavy burden of calcification on noninvasive imaging should alert the interventionist about underlying atherosclerosis, in which case angioplasty and/or stenting may be indicated (▶ Fig. 7.4).

7.2 Technique and Key Steps

- Because of high clot burden often encountered during such cases, we often choose guide catheters, aspiration catheters, and an SR with the largest possible profile.
- Aspiration through a balloon guide catheter (BGC) alone, with the balloon inflated, can be attempted (▶ Fig. 7.5). This simple setup occasionally results in successful clot extraction and complete recanalization, especially if the BGC can be delivered close to the occlusion.

- Modern guide catheters with improved trackability allow access to the ICA-T occlusion directly for direct aspiration thrombectomy (▶ Fig. 7.6) or in combination with an SR (▶ Fig. 7.7). For SR thrombectomy, we select an SR with the largest dimensions, such as a 6-mm × 40-mm Solitaire (Medtronic) or a 5-mm × 33-mm EmboTrap (Cerenovus).

7.3 Pearls and Pitfalls

- Large ICA clots can result in corking the tip of the guide catheter when the aspiration catheter and SR are withdrawn. This is indicated by the lack of blood return from the guide catheter. In such cases, injection through the guide catheter should not be performed. Rather, as continuous aspiration is applied to the guide catheter, we carefully remove the guide catheter completely and flush it with saline on the table. Thus, we prefer using a short 8–9 French (F) femoral sheath, depending on the type of guide catheter used (▶ Fig. 7.5, ▶ Fig. 7.6, ▶ Fig. 7.7) so that arterial access can be easily re-established, rather than going "sheathless" with a guide catheter.

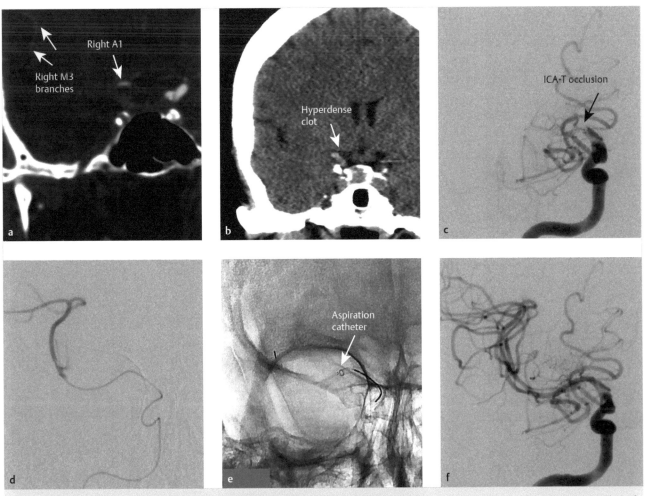

Fig. 7.3 Estimating clot length on digital subtraction angiography (DSA). **(a)** Computed tomography angiography (CTA), coronal view, showing lack of contrast material in the right internal carotid artery (ICA) intracranially. The right A1 is patent (*white arrow*). Distal M3 branches can be appreciated, but how far the clot extends into the middle cerebral artery (MCA) is difficult to determine (*yellow arrows*). **(b)** Noncontrast computed tomography (CT), coronal view, with a hyperdense clot sign (*arrow*). **(c)** DSA, anteroposterior (AP) view, confirming internal carotid artery terminus (ICA-T) occlusion on the right side (*arrow*). **(d)** Superselective microcatheter injection after traversing the right M1 occlusion. **(e)** Fluoroscopy showing deployed stent retriever (SR) (5-mm × 33-mm EmboTrap [Cerenovus]). An aspiration catheter (Jet 7 [Penumbra]) is seen pinning the proximal end of the clot (*arrow*). **(f)** DSA, AP view, post-thrombectomy.

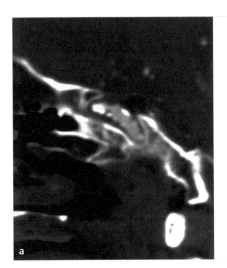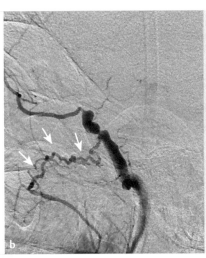

Fig. 7.4 Example of heavy calcifications at occlusion site. **(a)** Computed tomography angiography (CTA), sagittal view, with evidence of extensive calcifications and ulcerated appearance of internal carotid artery (ICA). **(b)** Digital subtraction angiography (DSA), lateral view, ICA injection, showing complete ICA occlusion just beyond the ophthalmic artery origin. Note an anastomosis of the cavernous ICA with internal maxillary branches of the external carotid artery (*arrows*). This angiographic appearance is highly suspicious of underlying atherosclerosis as the cause of ICA occlusion.

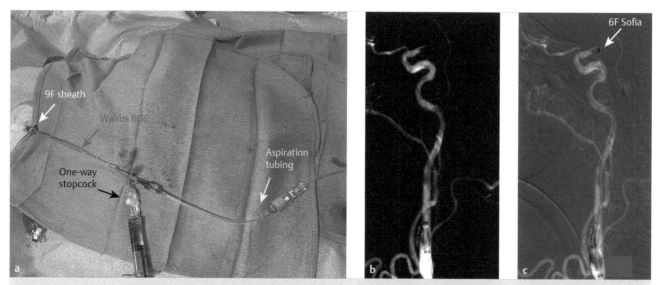

Fig. 7.5 Aspiration through a balloon guide catheter (BGC) alone followed by use of an aspiration catheter. **(a)** Photograph of procedural setup. A Walrus BGC (Q'Apel Medical) is used (*red arrow*). Once the balloon is inflated (*black arrow* points to one-way stopcock connecting a syringe with 50/50% contrast), aspiration can be turned on (*yellow arrow* points to aspiration tubing directly connected to the guide catheter). **(b)** Roadmap, lateral view, showing Walrus BGC in the cervical internal carotid artery (ICA). To optimize aspiration power, the balloon needs to be positioned higher. *Arrow* points to the internal carotid artery terminus (ICA-T) occlusion. If unsuccessful, as in this case, aspiration alone or stent retriever (SR) thrombectomy in conjunction with aspiration can be attempted next. Walrus BGC will accommodate most modern aspiration catheters given its 0.087-inch internal diameter. **(c)** Roadmap, lateral view, with 6F Sofia (MicroVention) catheter now accessing the clot (*arrow*). Aspiration thrombectomy is performed.

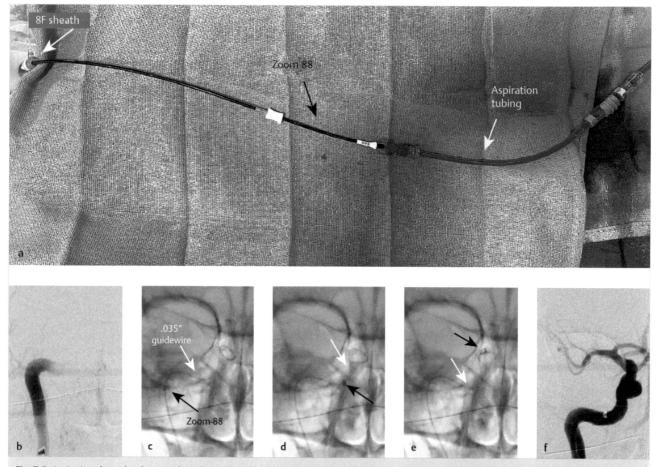

Fig. 7.6 Aspiration through a long guide catheter alone. **(a)** Photograph of procedural setup. Zoom 88 (*black arrow* [Imperative Care]) is a 0.088-inch 110-cm-long guide catheter capable of reaching the intracranial internal carotid artery (ICA) segments. An 8F short femoral sheath is used (*white arrow*). The guide is directly connected to aspiration tubing (*yellow arrow*). **(b)** Digital subtraction angiography (DSA), anteroposterior (AP) view, baseline angiographic run through the guide catheter, showing gradual tapering of contrast. **(c–e)** Fluoroscopy, sequential AP views, demonstrating tracking of Zoom 88 guide over an 0.035-inch guidewire (*white arrow*, Glidewire [Terumo]) until the operator feels resistance at the tip of the guide catheter, indicating that the catheter reached the clot. **(f)** DSA, AP view, postaspiration thrombectomy run. Patency of the right ICA and its branches is achieved.

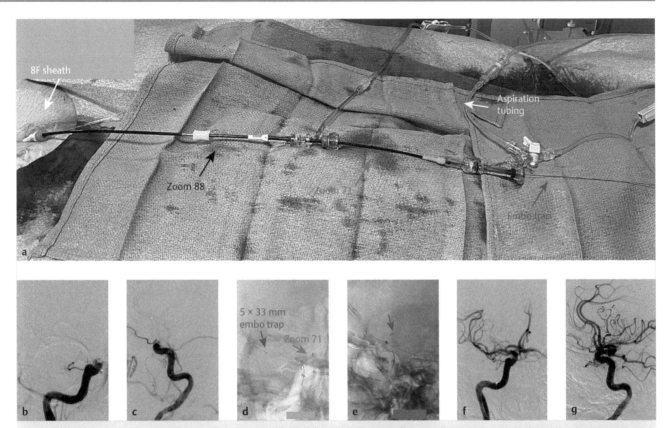

Fig. 7.7 Stent retriever (SR) thrombectomy in conjunction with aspiration. **(a)** Photograph of procedural setup. Zoom 88 (*black arrow*, Imperative Care) guide catheter, Zoom 71 (*red arrow*, Imperative Care) and EmboTrap SR pusher wire (*purple arrow*, Cerenovus) are shown. An 8F short femoral sheath is used (*white arrow*). The aspiration tubing (*yellow line*) is connected to the aspiration catheter. Digital subtraction angiography (DSA), **(b)** anteroposterior (AP), and **(c)** lateral views, baseline run, demonstrating internal carotid artery (ICA) occlusion just distal to the ophthalmic artery. Fluoroscopy, **(d)** AP and **(e)** lateral views, showing the radiopaque distal marker of 5-mm × 33-mm EmboTrap (*purple arrow*). Zoom 71 aspiration catheter is trapping the clot proximally (*red arrow*). DSA, **(f)** AP, and **(g)** lateral views, post-thrombectomy run. After two passes, successful reperfusion is achieved.

7.4 Cases with Videos and Images

7.4.1 Case 7.1 Balloon Guide Catheter and Stent Retriever

A patient with sudden onset of right hemiparesis and aphasia, National Institutes of Health Stroke Scale score > 20. Intracranial internal carotid artery (ICA) occlusion is suspected (▶ **Video 7.1;** ▶ Fig. 7.8, ▶ Fig. 7.9, ▶ Fig. 7.10, ▶ Fig. 7.11, ▶ Fig. 7.12).

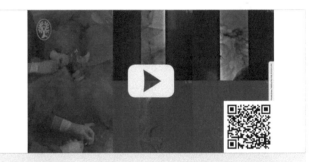

Video 7.1 Balloon Guide Catheter and Stent Retriever.

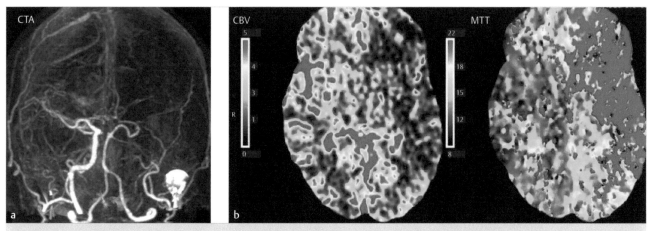

Fig. 7.8 Baseline noninvasive imaging. (a) Computed tomography angiography (CTA), three-dimensional (3D) reconstruction, showing lack of left internal carotid artery (ICA) opacification with contrast enhancement. (b) CT perfusion (CTP) images show the left hemisphere at risk: decreased cerebral blood volume (CBV; left) and prolonged mean transit time (MTT; right). Even with such an unfavorable imaging profile, there might still be benefit of thrombectomy, given the very poor natural history of such a large vessel occlusion if left untreated.

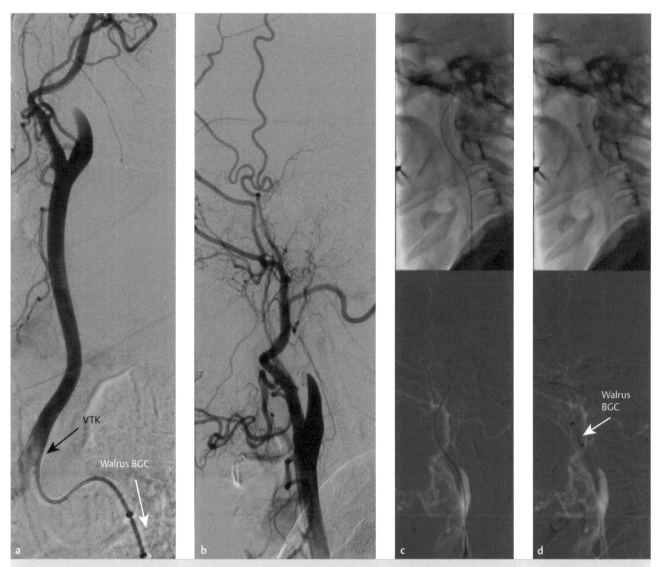

Fig. 7.9 Establishing access into the left internal carotid artery (ICA). (a,b) Digital subtraction angiography (DSA), sequential lateral views, left common carotid artery (CCA) injection, showing left ICA occlusion. There is gradual tapering of the contrast material, suggesting that the occlusion is located more distally within the left ICA than can be appreciated on angiography. The *black arrow* points to a 5F VTK catheter (Cook Medical) used to establish access into the left CCA and help navigate the balloon guide catheter (BGC) (*white arrow*, Walrus [Q'Apel Medical]). (c,d) Fluoroscopy (top images) and roadmap (bottom images), lateral views, showing delivery of the BGC (*white arrow*) over a 0.035-inch guidewire (GlideWire [Terumo]) and the VTK catheter into the cervical ICA.

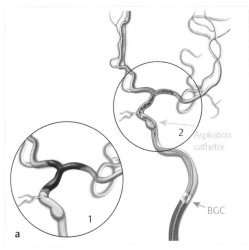
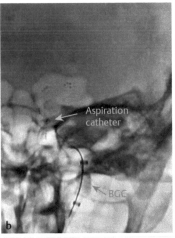

Fig. 7.10 **(a)** Artist's illustration of internal carotid artery terminus (ICA-T) thrombectomy using a balloon guide catheter (BGC) and a stent retriever (SR). In step 1, a large clot in the ICA-T extending into the left middle cerebral artery (MCA) and anterior cerebral artery (ACA) can be appreciated. In step 2, inflation of the BGC (*blue arrow*) arrests flow, thus preventing dislodgment of the clot that is trapped by the SR device and aspiration catheter (*green arrow*). **(b)** Fluoroscopy, anteroposterior (AP) view, from the corresponding clinical case. (**a**: © Thieme/Jennifer Pryll)

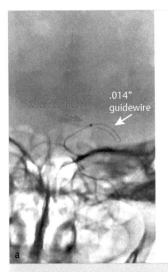
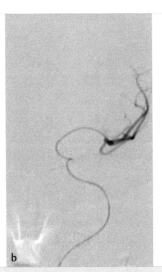
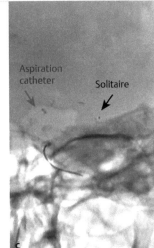
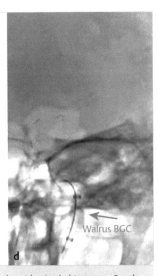

Fig. 7.11 Stent retriever (SR) thrombectomy is performed. **(a)** Fluoroscopy, working projection, showing a 0.014-inch guidewire (*white arrow*, Synchro [Stryker]) and microcatheter (*red arrow*, Velocity [Penumbra]) traversing the clot. Creating a loop at the microwire tip is a safe way to navigate through the occlusion and avoid vessel perforation. **(b)** Digital subtraction angiography (DSA), superselective injection through the microcatheter, confirming its positioning within a distal middle cerebral artery (MCA) branch. **(c)** Fluoroscopy, showing the aspiration catheter (*green arrow*, 6F Sofia, MicroVention) and 6-mm × 40-mm Solitaire SR (*black arrow*, Medtronic). **(d)** Fluoroscopy, showing inflated balloon of the Walrus balloon guide catheter (BGC) (*blue arrow*, Q'Apel Medical) as thrombectomy is performed with the SR in conjunction with aspiration through the Sofia catheter.

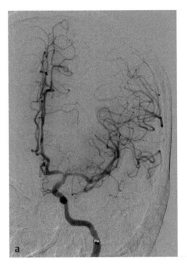
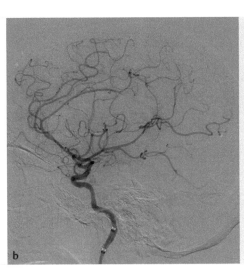

Fig. 7.12 Digital subtraction angiography (DSA) after thrombectomy. DSA, **(a)** anteroposterior (AP), and **(b)** lateral views, showing thrombolysis in cerebral infarction (TICI) 3 reperfusion.

7.4.2 Case 7.2 Intracranial Stenting

This patient with a known chronic left internal carotid artery (ICA) occlusion is admitted with acute stroke secondary to flow-limiting right ICA intracranial stenosis (▶ Video 7.2; ▶ Fig. 7.13, ▶ Fig. 7.14, ▶ Fig. 7.15, ▶ Fig. 7.16).

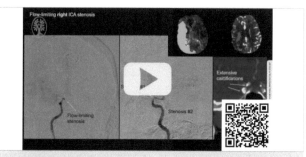

Video 7.2 Intracranial Stenting.

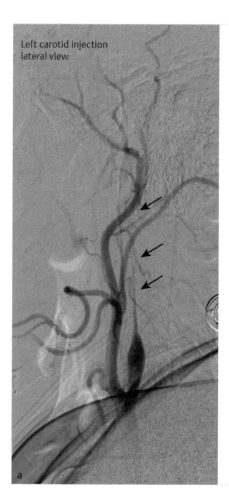

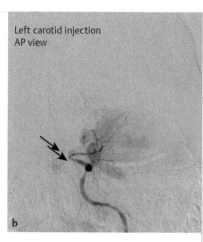

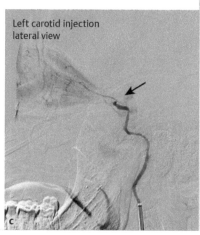

Fig. 7.13 Left carotid artery baseline digital subtraction angiography (DSA). (a) DSA, left common carotid artery (CCA) injection, lateral cervical view, showing greatly diminished flow through the left internal carotid artery (ICA) (arrows). (b) DSA, left CCA injection, anteroposterior (AP) view, and (c) lateral intracranial view, demonstrating complete left ICA occlusion intracranially (arrows).

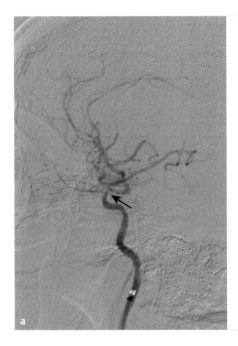
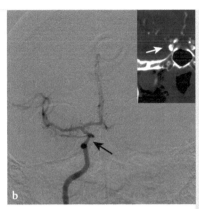
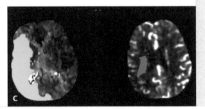

Fig. 7.14 Right carotid artery baseline digital subtraction angiography (DSA). **(a)** DSA, right internal carotid artery (ICA) injection, lateral view, and **(b)** anteroposterior (AP) view, showing diminished intracranial flow. The *arrows* point to intracranial stenosis. The insert in **(b)** is a coronal computed tomography angiography (CTA) view showing extensive calcifications of the intracranial ICA at the area of stenosis (*arrow*). **(c)** CT perfusion (CTP) images confirming a large perfusion deficit in the right hemisphere. *Green*—tissue at risk; *red*—small ischemic core.

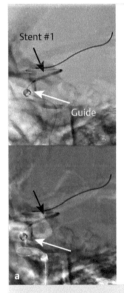
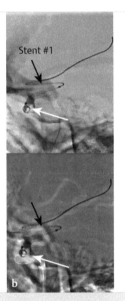
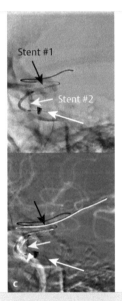
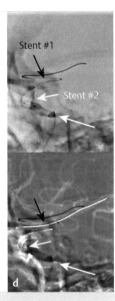
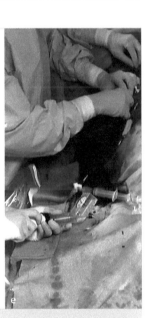

Fig. 7.15 Steps of internal carotid artery (ICA) intracranial stenting. **(a)** Fluoroscopy (top images) and **(b)** roadmap (bottom images) views showing the first balloon-mounted stent (*black arrow*, 3-mm × 15-mm Resolute Onyx [Medtronic]) being delivered and deployed. These coronary stents offer excellent radial force but are hard to deliver through cerebral tortuosity; thus, two shorter Resolute Onyx stents, rather than one long stent, are chosen in this case. Also note the close proximity of the guide catheter (*white arrows*, TracStar [Imperative Care]) to the area of stenosis to help tracking the device. **(c)** Fluoroscopy (top images) and **(d)** roadmap (bottom images) views showing delivery and deployment of the second 3-mm × 15-mm Resolute Onyx stent (*yellow arrows*) to partially overlap with the first stent. **(e)** Photograph, showing the operator holding the stent while gradually inflating the balloon using an inflation device. Gradual slow inflation by 1 atmosphere every 30 to 60 seconds is performed in such cases.

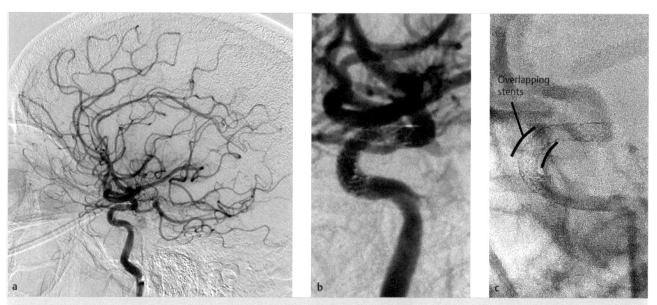

Fig. 7.16 Digital subtraction angiography (DSA) after internal carotid artery (ICA) stenting. **(a)** DSA, lateral view, standard magnification, and **(b)** high magnification, showing greatly improved intracranial flow. **(c)** Fluoroscopy, lateral view, of the two-stent construct. The region where the two stents overlap is indicated by the black lines.

8 Tandem Occlusion

General Description

Tandem occlusion in acute stroke typically presents as an occlusion or nearly occlusive flow-limiting lesion of the extracranial (often, cervical) portion of the internal carotid artery (ICA) with concomitant more distal occlusion of intracranial ICA or its distal branches (mainly, the middle cerebral artery [MCA]). Such a lesion is a major challenge for thrombectomy in acute anterior circulation strokes; the cases tend to be longer, often requiring the use of multiple catheters and devices, with angiographic and clinical outcomes worse than in isolated ICA terminus or MCA occlusions. Management options for posterior circulation strokes resulting from tandem occlusion are discussed in a separate chapter.

Keywords: Angioplasty, stenting, carotid occlusion, thrombectomy

8.1 Anatomical and Imaging Aspects

- The main treatment approach to this challenging category of patients can be broken down into two categories:
  - The "Neck-first" approach: treatment of the cervical lesion with angioplasty and/or stenting followed by intracranial thrombectomy.
  - The "Head-first" approach: Performing thrombectomy first by traversing the cervical lesion with a guide catheter. Treatment of the cervical lesion is addressed after intracranial recanalization is achieved.
- Such a binary way of thinking when performing treatment is not always applicable, and a simple recipe that fits all patients does not exist. For example, a case of severely calcified ICA stenosis may require angioplasty of the cervical lesion to deliver the guide catheter for intracranial thrombectomy, followed by stenting (neck-first, head-next, neck-last); this is just one scenario in which an individualized approach is required.
- Careful examination of the baseline imaging helps the interventionist recognize the underlying etiology and composition of the cervical lesion (chronicity, morphology, and severity of atherosclerotic plaque [▶ Fig. 8.1], underlying dissection, presence of intraluminal thrombus [▶ Fig. 8.2]), which in turn will dictate the ease and risk of traversing this lesion.
- When determining the treatment strategy for the neck lesion (angioplasty alone vs. stenting), the extent of the ischemic core burden on noncontrast computed tomography (CT; ▶ Fig. 8.3) or perfusion imaging and the angiographic appearance of residual ICA stenosis (▶ Fig. 8.4) are used to estimate the likelihood of hemorrhagic transformation and risk for early ICA reocclusion.

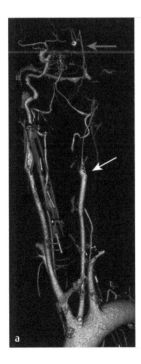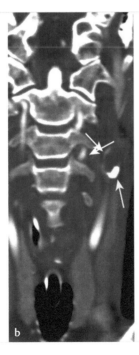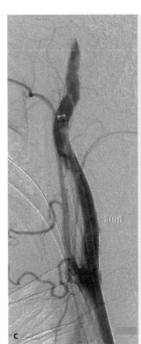

Fig. 8.1 Tandem lesion with soft plaque at the internal carotid artery (ICA) bifurcation. (a) Computed tomography angiogram (CTA), three-dimensional (3D) reconstruction, showing left ICA origin occlusion (*white arrow*) and tandem intracranial occlusion (*red arrow*). (b) CTA, coronal view, showing the complex nature of the ICA origin plaque. Calcifications are present (*yellow arrow*). However, most of the plaque consists of noncalcified soft components (*white arrows*), which are prone to distal embolization. In such cases, securing the plaque with a stent before traversing this lesion with a guide catheter is necessary. (c) Digital subtraction angiogram (DSA), lateral view. Once the plaque was secured with stenting (Wallstent [Boston Scientific], an 0.088-inch guide catheter (Neuron Max [Penumbra]) was delivered through the stent, and thrombectomy of the intracranial lesion was performed.

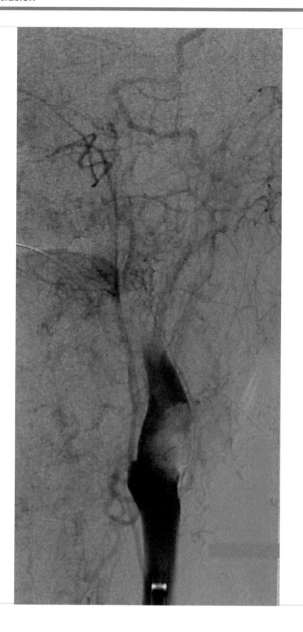

Fig. 8.2 Intraluminal thrombus at the carotid bifurcation. Digital subtraction angiogram (DSA), anteroposterior (AP) view, showing a large mass (fresh thrombus) at the carotid bifurcation, causing near-complete internal carotid artery (ICA) origin occlusion. Unless stented, such an unstable lesion is at risk of major distal embolization when crossed by a guide catheter.

8.2 Technique and Key Steps

- The use of a combination of a balloon guide catheter (BGC) and a distal filter minimizes the risk of embolic complications and is reasonable to consider in cases with soft plaque (▶ Fig. 8.5) or an intraluminal clot component.
- A Mo.Ma proximal cerebral protection device (Medtronic) provides total flow arrest by occluding both the external carotid artery and common carotid artery (CCA), whereas BGCs occlude only the CCA (Chapter 5 "Internal Carotid Artery Occlusion"). However, the Mo.Ma device is not designed for intracranial thrombectomy. The device will not track through the stent, and its inner diameter is too small to accommodate aspiration catheters. If the Mo.Ma device is used for ICA stenting, it needs to be exchanged for a guide catheter to address the intracranial lesion. Thus, the Mo.Ma is rarely used for acute stroke interventions.

8.3 Pearls and Pitfalls

- If the cervical lesion is treated with carotid stent placement and a stent retriever (SR) is used for the treatment of the intracranial lesion, we carefully advance the guide catheter beyond the distal end of the freshly placed stent. This is to ensure that the SR and carotid stent do become entangled during clot retrieval.

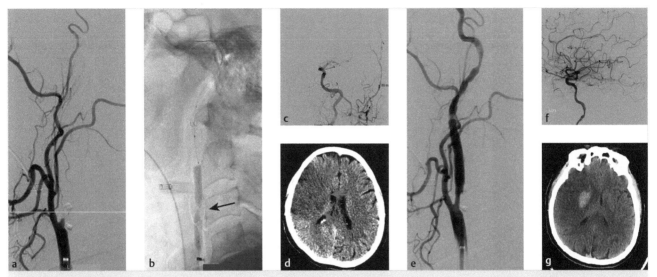

Fig. 8.3 Tandem internal carotid artery (ICA) occlusion: emergent stenting is high risk. **(a)** Digital subtraction angiogram (DSA), lateral view, right ICA injection, showing ICA origin occlusion. **(b)** Roadmap showing balloon angioplasty. Note the "waist" in the midportion of the balloon (*arrow*, 4-mm × 40-mm Aviator [Cardinal Health]), indicating the maximal area of stenosis with underlying calcification. Several rounds of angioplasty were performed. **(c)** DSA, anteroposterior (AP) view. Tandem intracranial ICA terminus occlusion is present. **(d)** Noncontrast head computed tomography (CT), axial view. Baseline CT already shows a large ischemic core (*arrows*), Alberta Stroke Program Early CT Score (ASPECTS)<6. **(e)** DSA, lateral view. Given the large ischemic core burden, no emergent stenting was performed in this case. **(f)** DSA, left ICA injection, post thrombectomy. Thrombolysis in cerebral infarction (TICI) grade 3 reperfusion is achieved. **(g)** Noncontrast head CT, repeated the following day. A small area of hemorrhagic transformation is seen within the right basal ganglia region. Stenting this patient emergently, with glycoprotein IIb/IIIa agents administered intraprocedurally and antiplatelet agents administered immediately postprocedure, would have likely worsened the degree of hemorrhagic transformation.

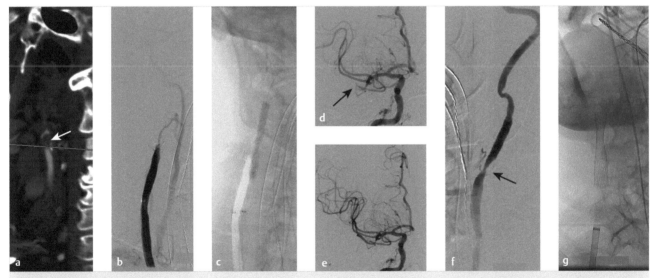

Fig. 8.4 Tandem internal carotid artery (ICA) occlusion: a safe case for stenting. **(a)** Computed tomography angiogram (CTA), axial view, showing occlusion of the right ICA origin (*arrow*). **(b)** Digital subtraction angiogram (DSA), anteroposterior (AP) view, confirming complete occlusion of the right ICA origin. **(c)** Roadmap, AP view. A 5-mm × 40-mm Aviator angioplasty balloon (Cardinal Health) is used. **(d)** DSA, intracranial view, showing a tandem inferior division right M2 occlusion (*arrow*). **(e)** DSA, showing successful aspiration thrombectomy of the right M2 occlusion. **(f)** DSA, cervical AP view, repeat right common carotid artery (CCA) injection. Severe residual stenosis is present at the carotid bifurcation (*arrow*). Angioplasty alone will likely result in early reocclusion; thus, emergent stenting is indicated. **(g)** Fluoroscopy, showing Xact stent (Abbott). The Xact is a laser-cut closed-cell stent with great radial force, which is an optimal choice for such a severely stenotic lesion.

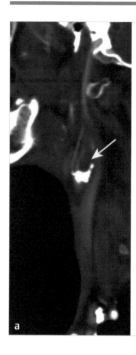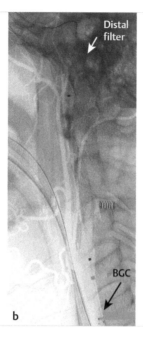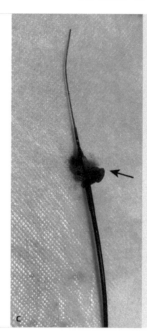

Fig. 8.5 Combining a balloon guide catheter (BGC) and a distal filter. **(a)** Computed tomography angiogram (CTA), lateral view. Soft plaque, possibly with adjacent fresh clot is appreciated (*arrow*). **(b)** Digital subtraction angiogram (DSA), lateral view, roadmap. An 8-French (F) BGC (Cello [Medtronic]) is positioned in the distal common carotid artery (CCA) (*black arrow*). A distal filter (Emboshield NAV6 [Abbott]) is deployed above the C1–C2 level (*white arrow*). **(c)** A thrombus (*arrow*) was captured by the distal filter.

8.4 Cases with Videos and Images

8.4.1 Case 8.1 Tandem CCA and MCA Lesion and Aspiration Thrombectomy

A patient with sudden onset of right hemiparesis, left gaze deviation, and aphasia (▶ **Video 8.1**; ▶ Fig. 8.6, ▶ Fig. 8.7, ▶ Fig. 8.8, ▶ Fig. 8.9, ▶ Fig. 8.10, ▶ Fig. 8.11).

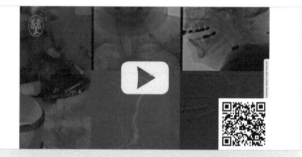

Video 8.1 Tandem CCA and MCA Lesion and Aspiration Thrombectomy.

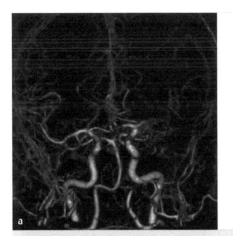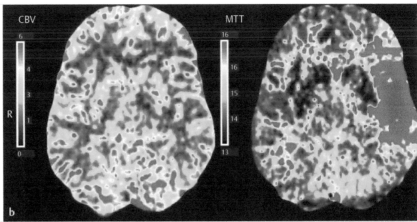

Fig. 8.6 Baseline noninvasive imaging. **(a)** Computed tomography angiogram (CTA), three-dimensional (3D) reconstruction, showing left M1 occlusion. **(b)** Computed tomography perfusion (CTP) images show the left hemisphere at risk: preserved cerebral blood volume (CBV; left) and prolonged mean transit time (MTT; right).

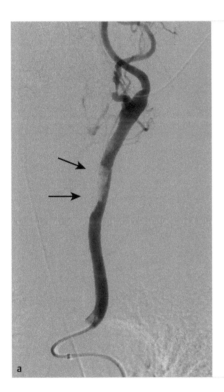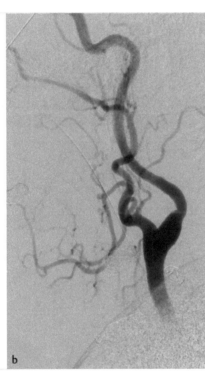

Fig. 8.7 Left common carotid artery (CCA) lesion. **(a)** Digital subtraction angiogram (DSA), anteroposterior (AP) view, left CCA injection, showing high-grade stenosis of the midportion of the left CCA (*arrows*). There is likely a superimposed fresh thrombus as well. **(b)** DSA, lateral view, left CCA injection. The carotid bifurcation is patent.

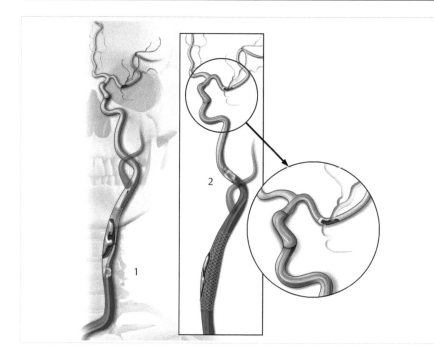

Fig. 8.8 Artist's illustration of the treatment of this case. In step 1, the high-risk left common carotid artery (CCA) lesion is treated first using a carotid stent. In step 2, intracranial middle cerebral artery (MCA) aspiration thrombectomy is performed. (© Thieme/Jennifer Pryll)

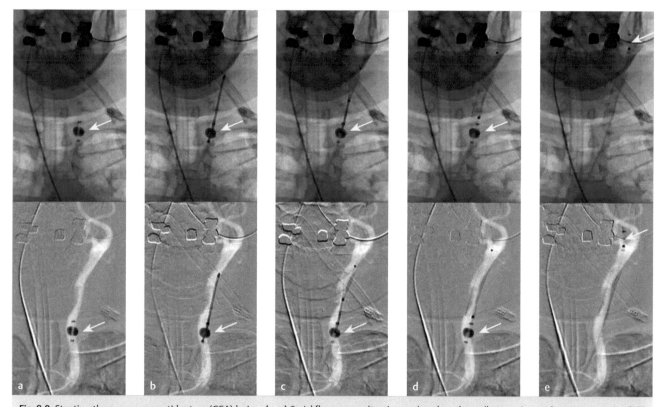

Fig. 8.9 Stenting the common carotid artery (CCA) lesion. **(a–e)** Serial fluoroscopy (top images) and roadmap (bottom images), anteroposterior (AP) views, showing a balloon guide catheter (BGC) (Walrus, Q'Apel Medical; *arrow* in each image) positioned in the left CCA proximal to the stenotic lesion. With the balloon inflated, a large diameter 10-mm carotid stent (Wallstent [Boston Scientific]) is delivered over an 0.014-inch guidewire (Spartacore [Abbott]) and deployed. The balloon is then deflated, and the guide catheter is advanced through the stent delivery system and into the left internal carotid artery (ICA) for intracranial thrombectomy before removing the guidewire.

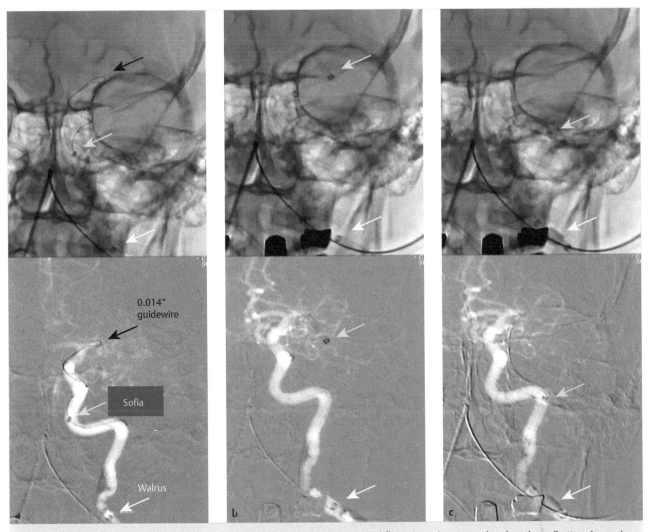

Fig. 8.10 Left middle cerebral artery (MCA) aspiration thrombectomy. **(a–c)** Sequential fluoroscopy (top images) and roadmap (bottom images), anteroposterior (AP) views, showing a balloon guide catheter (BGC) (*yellow arrows*, Walrus, Q'Apel Medical; *arrow* in each image) now positioned in the left ICA. The aspiration catheter (*green arrows*, 6F Sofia [MicroVention]) is delivered over an 0.014-inch guidewire (*black arrows* in **a**, Synchro [Stryker]) and 0.025-inch microcatheter (*blue arrows* in **a**, Velocity [Penumbra]). Note in **(c)** inflation of the BGC when withdrawing the aspiration catheter.

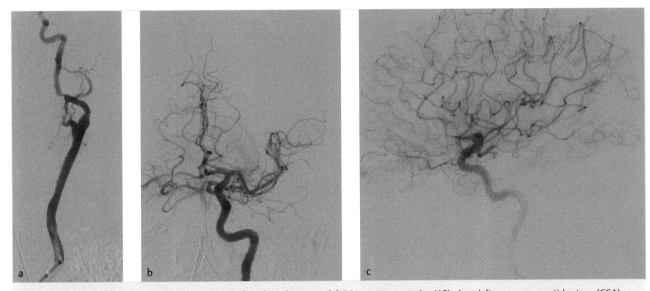

Fig. 8.11 Final digital subtraction angiogram (DSA) after thrombectomy. **(a)** DSA, anteroposterior (AP) view, left common carotid artery (CCA) injection, showing patent left CCA after stent placement. **(b)** DSA, AP view and **(c)** lateral view, showing fully patent left middle cerebral artery (MCA) with thrombolysis in cerebral infarction (TICI) 3 reperfusion.

8.4.2 Case 8.2 Tandem ICA Occlusion and Stent Retriever Thrombectomy

A patient is admitted to the emergency department globally aphasic, with right hemiparesis and right hemianopsia (▶ **Video 8.2**; ▶ Fig. 8.12, ▶ Fig. 8.13, ▶ Fig. 8.14, ▶ Fig. 8.15, ▶ Fig. 8.16, ▶ Fig. 8.17).

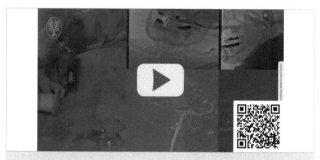

Video 8.2 Tandem ICA Occlusion and Stent Retriever Thrombectomy.

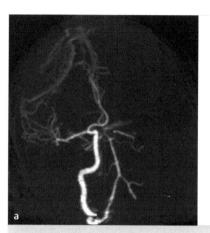
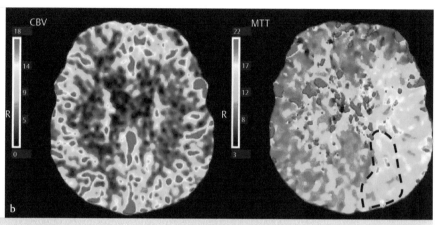

Fig. 8.12 Baseline noninvasive imaging. **(a)** Computed tomography angiogram (CTA), three-dimensional (3D) reconstruction, showing loss of contrast signal in the left internal carotid artery (ICA) and middle cerebral artery (MCA). **(b)** Computed tomography perfusion (CTP) images show the left hemisphere at risk: preserved cerebral blood volume (CBV) (left) and prolonged mean transit time (MTT) (right). The left posterior cerebral artery (PCA) territory is also affected (outlined area), indicating that the patient likely has a "fetal"-type PCA anatomical variant.

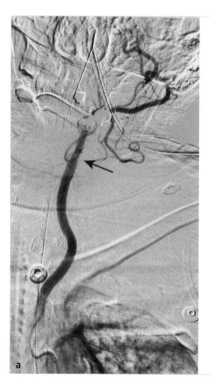
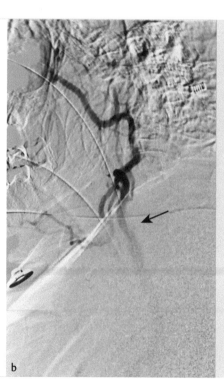

Fig. 8.13 Left internal carotid artery (ICA) origin occlusion. **(a)** Digital subtraction angiogram (DSA), anteroposterior (AP) and **(b)** lateral views, left common carotid artery (CCA) injection, showing occlusion of the ICA at the bifurcation (*arrow* in each image).

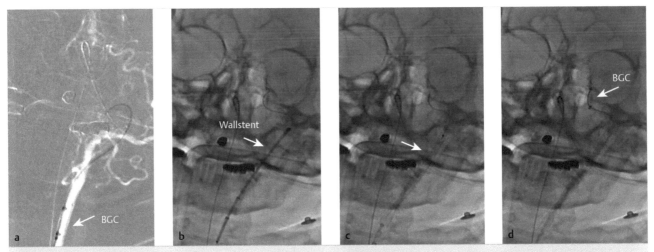

Fig. 8.14 Stenting the internal carotid artery (ICA) lesion. **(a)** Roadmap, left common carotid artery (CCA) injection, anteroposterior (AP) view, showing a balloon guide catheter (BGC) (*arrow*, Walrus [Q'Apel Medical]). placed in the distal part of the left CCA. **(b)** Fluoroscopy, AP view, showing a carotid stent (*arrow*, Wallstent [Boston Scientific]) being delivered over an 0.014-inch guidewire (Spartacore [Abbott]). **(c)** Fluoroscopy, AP view. The Wallstent has been deployed (*arrow*). **(d)** Fluoroscopy, AP view, showing the BGC (*arrow*) now advanced through the stent into the cervical ICA segment.

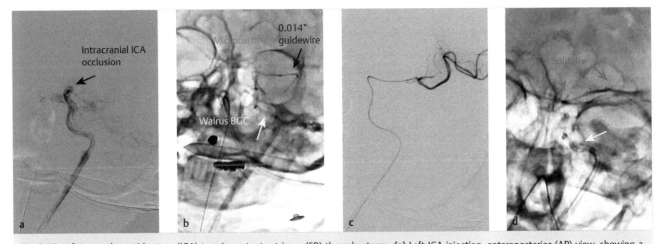

Fig. 8.15 Left internal carotid artery (ICA) terminus stent retriever (SR) thrombectomy. **(a)** Left ICA injection, anteroposterior (AP) view, showing a tandem left ICA terminus occlusion (*arrow*). **(b)** Fluoroscopy, AP view, showing a balloon guide catheter (BGC) (*yellow arrow*, Walrus [Q'Apel Medical]) in the petrous ICA segment. A 0.025-inch microcatheter (*blue arrow*, Velocity [Penumbra]) and 0.014-inch guidewire (*black arrow*, Synchro [Stryker]) are used to cross the thrombus. **(c)** Digital subtraction angiogram (DSA), superselective injection through the microcatheter, confirming its safe position prior to SR delivery and deployment. **(d)** Fluoroscopy, anteroposterior (AP) view, showing SR thrombectomy. A 6-mm × 40-mm Solitaire (*red arrows*, Medtronic) is retrieved with the balloon (*yellow arrow*) now inflated for proximal flow arrest.

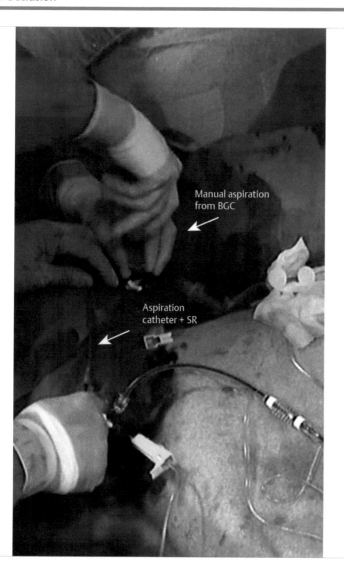

Fig. 8.16 Stent retriever (SR) thrombectomy with a balloon guide catheter (BGC). Photograph showing one operator aspirating from the BGC (*white arrow*) while the second operator is retrieving the SR and aspiration catheter (*yellow arrow*).

Manual aspiration from BGC

Aspiration catheter + SR

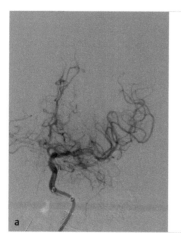

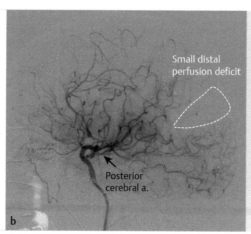

Small distal perfusion deficit

Posterior cerebral a.

Fig. 8.17 Final digital subtraction angiogram (DSA) after thrombectomy. DSA, left internal carotid artery (ICA) injection, **(a)** anteroposterior (AP) and **(b)** lateral views, showing a small distal perfusion deficit (outlined area) but otherwise patent left middle cerebral artery (MCA) corresponding to thrombolysis in cerebral infarction (TICI) 2C reperfusion. Note robust opacification of the left posterior cerebral artery (PCA) (*arrow*), confirming our suspicion that the left PCA was affected by the intracranial occlusion seen on baseline computed tomography perfusion (CTP) imaging in ▶ Fig. 8.12b.

9 Proximal Middle Cerebral Artery Occlusion—Stent-Retriever Thrombectomy

General Description

Stent-retriever (SR) thrombectomy is a common first-line approach to mechanical thrombectomy for large vessel occlusion (LVO). This technique revolutionized the field of acute stroke interventions after several independent randomized trials published in 2015 demonstrated the safety and efficacy of this treatment over medical management alone in patients with LVO. Proximal middle cerebral artery (MCA) occlusion was the most common LVO location in these trials. SR devices are temporarily deployed and then withdrawn after capture and removal of the thrombus. A variety of techniques and modifications to this thrombectomy approach currently exist for the treatment of proximal MCA, which is the focus of this chapter.

Keywords: Balloon guide catheter, middle cerebral artery, stent retriever, thrombectomy

9.1 Anatomical and Imaging Aspects

- The anatomy of the MCA is highly variable. Recognizing its variations ensures safe performance of the thrombectomy procedure and accurate interpretation of procedural outcomes (▶ Fig. 9.1, ▶ Fig. 9.2). There is no uniform agreement on the preferred classification of MCA segments for the purpose of endovascular therapy (EVT)—whether grading should be done according to the order of branching segments, by direction of the segments (horizontally—M1; vertically along the operculum—M2; horizontally in the Sylvian fissure—M3), or by supply territory.
- Unlike contact aspiration thrombectomy alone, where only visualization of the proximal end of the clot is needed to perform clot extraction, a more detailed understanding

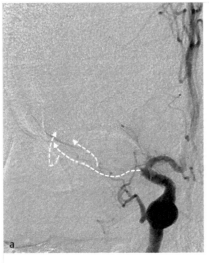
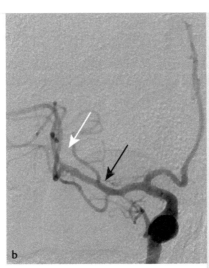
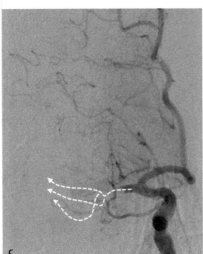
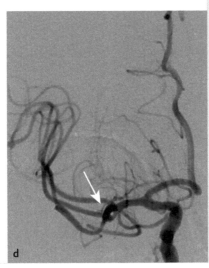

Fig. 9.1 Examples of variations in proximal middle cerebral artery (MCA) anatomy. **(a)** Digital subtraction angiogram (DSA), anteroposterior (AP) view, right internal carotid artery (ICA) injection, showing M1 origin occlusion. The *white dashed line* shows the most likely direction of the guidewire route, especially if a J-type shape is used. The *yellow dashed lines* correspond to alternative routes that can also occur. Because occlusions are crossed "blindly," familiarity with MCA variants may help the neurointerventionists recognize and prevent guidewire perforation. **(b)** Upon revascularization, this patient is found to have a rather long horizontal segment of the MCA (*white arrow*). Alternatively, one could argue that the bifurcation point is more proximal (*black arrow*), and this patient has an MCA trifurcation with one of the M2 branches (*white arrow*) disproportionally larger than the other two. Such anatomical challenges often become relevant when classifying cases for clinical trial results interpretations. **(c)** Digital subtraction angiogram (DSA), AP view, right ICA injection, showing proximal M1 occlusion. The *dashed lines* show the number of different routes the guidewire may take when traversing the occlusion. **(d)** Upon recanalization, it becomes clear that this patient has a rather short M1 horizontal segment (*arrow*) before it trifurcates.

of clot morphology is needed when SR thrombectomy is performed. Ideally, the SR should be oversized, extending by at least one-third of its length beyond the distal end of the clot (▶ Fig. 9.3). This ensures that as the SR is pulled back (retrieved), if any rolling of the clot occurs along the device, the distal end of the SR will be able to prevent clot breakdown and embolization. Many operators also advocate oversizing the SR diameter; as the stent is stretched during thrombectomy, its diameter can be reduced.

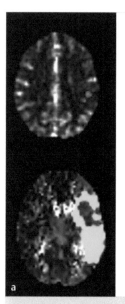
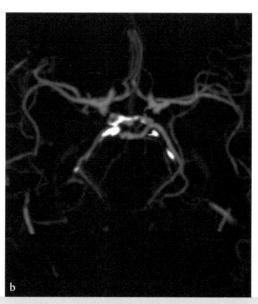
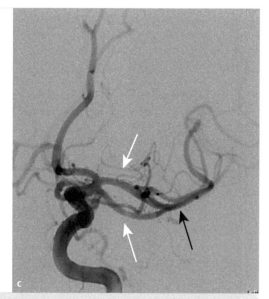

Fig. 9.2 An example of middle cerebral artery (MCA) duplication. **(a)** CT perfusion (CTP) image showing a large, left MCA perfusion deficit (top image—stroke core, bottom image—ischemic penumbra). **(b)** Computed tomographic angiography (CTA) appears to show patent intracranial vessels. However, because of the perfusion deficit and corresponding symptoms suggestive of left hemispheric syndrome, the patient is immediately taken for angiography. **(c)** Digital subtraction angiogram (DSA), anteroposterior (AP) view, showing two MCA trunks (*white arrows*). One of these trunks has a proximal occlusion (*black arrow*), which explains the perfusion and clinical findings.

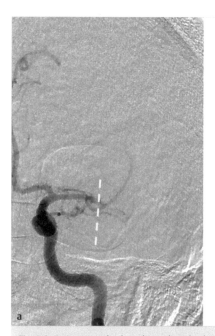
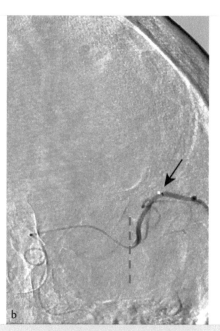
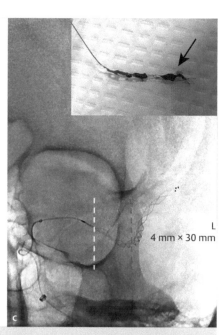

Fig. 9.3 Estimating clot length on digital subtraction angiogram (DSA). **(a)** DSA, anteroposterior (AP) view, showing distal left M1 occlusion. The *dashed line* indicates the proximal end of the clot. This patient has poor leptomeningeal collaterals, and the distal end of the clot cannot be visualized angiographically. **(b)** Superselective microcatheter injection after traversing the left M1 occlusion. Retrograde filling of contrast material stops at the distal end of the clot (*red dashed line*). The *black arrow* points to the tip of the microcatheter. **(c)** Fluoroscopy showing deployed stent retriever (SR) (Trevo [Stryker]). The device is optimally positioned, allowing plenty of extra length of the device distal to the clot. The proximal and distal end of the clot is shown with *yellow* and *red dashed lines*. If clot breakdown occurs during SR retrieval, this extra device length will minimize the risk of distal embolization by capturing and retrieving clot debris. The inset photograph shows that despite clot "rolling" encountered during thrombectomy (*arrow*), the device captured the clot more distally.

• The distal end of the clot is often easy to visualize on computed tomographic angiography (CTA) in patients with robust collaterals because of backfilling of iodine contrast material into the M2 or M3 branches and opacifying the vessel distally (▶ Fig. 9.4). However, in patients with poor collaterals, often only the proximal end of the clot can be detected. A superselective injection through a microcatheter can also help determine the distal end of the clot once the occlusion is traversed and the guidewire is removed. This also ensures the microcatheter's position inside the vessel and confirms that no vessel perforation has occurred (▶ Fig. 9.5). If contrast extravasation is suspected, cone beam computed tomography (CT) can be performed immediately in the angiography suite.

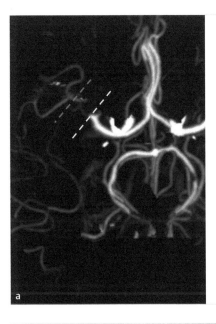
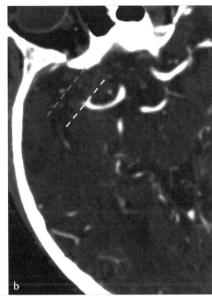

Fig. 9.4 Estimating clot length on computed tomographic angiography (CTA). **(a)** Three-dimensional (3D) reconstruction showing a filling defect of the proximal right middle cerebral artery (MCA), indicating the proximal and distal end of the clot (*yellow* and *red dashed lines*, respectively). **(b)** Axial view, filling defect within the distal right M1 segment pointing to the location of the clot (the *yellow* and *red dashed lines* correspond to the proximal and distal ends of the clot, respectively).

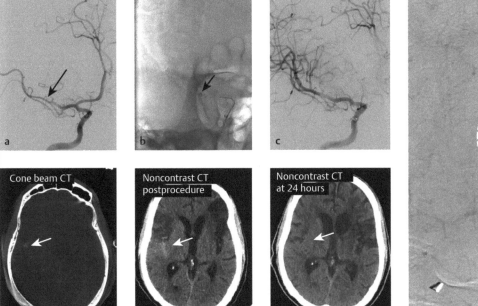

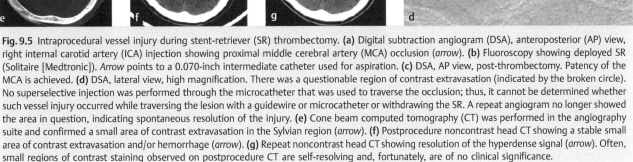

Fig. 9.5 Intraprocedural vessel injury during stent-retriever (SR) thrombectomy. **(a)** Digital subtraction angiogram (DSA), anteroposterior (AP) view, right internal carotid artery (ICA) injection showing proximal middle cerebral artery (MCA) occlusion (*arrow*). **(b)** Fluoroscopy showing deployed SR (Solitaire [Medtronic]). *Arrow* points to a 0.070-inch intermediate catheter used for aspiration. **(c)** DSA, AP view, post-thrombectomy. Patency of the MCA is achieved. **(d)** DSA, lateral view, high magnification. There was a questionable region of contrast extravasation (indicated by the broken circle). No superselective injection was performed through the microcatheter that was used to traverse the occlusion; thus, it cannot be determined whether such vessel injury occurred while traversing the lesion with a guidewire or microcatheter or withdrawing the SR. A repeat angiogram no longer showed the area in question, indicating spontaneous resolution of the injury. **(e)** Cone beam computed tomography (CT) was performed in the angiography suite and confirmed a small area of contrast extravasation in the Sylvian region (*arrow*). **(f)** Postprocedure noncontrast head CT showing a stable small area of contrast extravasation and/or hemorrhage (*arrow*). **(g)** Repeat noncontrast head CT showing resolution of the hyperdense signal (*arrow*). Often, small regions of contrast staining observed on postprocedure CT are self-resolving and, fortunately, are of no clinical significance.

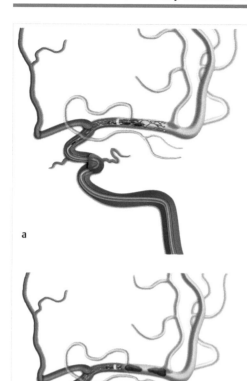

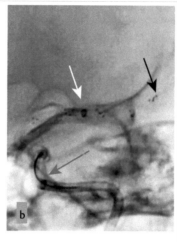

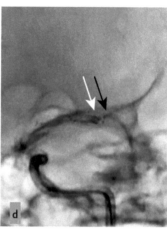

Fig. 9.6 Stent-retriever (SR) thrombectomy in conjunction with continuous aspiration. (a) Artist's illustration showing ideal capture of clot by an SR and aspiration catheter. The aspiration catheter (in *green*) engages only the proximal end of the clot for additional efficacy. (b) Fluoroscopy showing the distal end of the aspiration catheter (*white arrow*) and the SR (Solitaire; *black arrow*). Both catheter and SR can now be pulled back into the long guide sheath (*red arrow*). (c) Artist's illustration demonstrating clot breakdown and embolization, which can occur when an SR is mistakenly completely pulled back into the aspiration catheter. If a large clot is encountered, such a maneuver can strip portions of the clot. (d) Fluoroscopy showing the distal tip of the aspiration catheter (*white arrow*) and SR (*black arrow*) nearly overlapping now. (a, c: © Thieme/ Jennifer Pryll)

9.2 Technique and Key Steps

- SR thrombectomy is commonly performed using the following types of access catheters: a balloon guide catheter (BGC), a long sheath plus an aspiration catheter, or both a BGC and an aspiration catheter in conjunction with an SR.
- For a combination aspiration catheter and SR approach to be effective, it is critical to ensure that the SR is not fully retracted into the aspiration catheter to prevent stripping of the clot (▶ Fig. 9.6). The operator will often feel a "catch" on the SR push wire, indicating that the aspiration catheter tip has engaged the proximal end of the clot (▶ Fig. 9.7). At this point, both the SR and aspiration catheter are withdrawn into the guide catheter as a single unit. The aspiration catheter at this point is usually connected to an aspiration pump, because using manual aspiration with a syringe and trying to pull the catheter and SR at the same time becomes technically cumbersome.
- Traversing the occlusion with a "J"-shaped tip of the guidewire ensures catheterization of the main vessel, rather than smaller side branches that are more prone to injury (▶ Fig. 9.8).

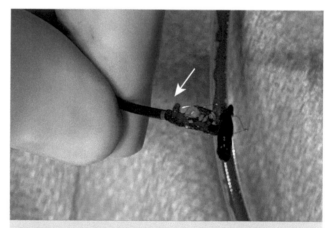

Fig. 9.7 Stent-retriever (SR) thrombectomy in conjunction with continuous aspiration. Photograph showing the aspiration catheter engaging the proximal end of the clot (*arrow*). The struts of the SR (Solitaire, [Medtronic]) are engaging the remainder of the clot.

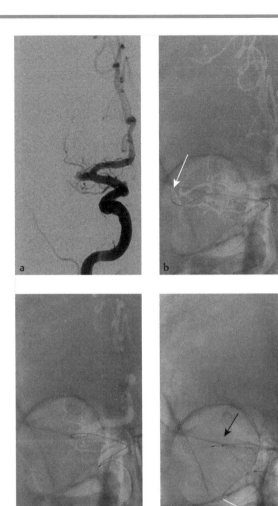
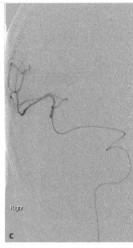
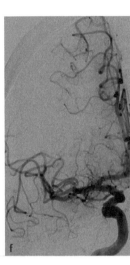

Fig. 9.8 Traversing the middle cerebral artery (MCA) occlusion. **(a)** Digital subtraction angiogram (DSA), anteroposterior (AP) view, right internal carotid artery (ICA) injection shows M1 occlusion. **(h)** Roadmap, demonstrating traversing the occlusion with a 0.014-inch guidewire (Synchro [Stryker]) with a nearly straight tip (*arrow*). **(c)** DSA, superselective injection through the microcatheter (Velocity [Penumbra]), shows no active contrast extravasation. However, note the small diameter of the MCA branch that is catheterized. **(d)** Roadmap showing another attempt to traverse the occlusion, this time with a "J"-shaped guidewire to ensure that the largest MCA branch is selected. **(e)** Fluoroscopy, showing a deployed stent retriever (SR) (Trevo [Stryker]). The *arrow* points to the distal tip of the microcatheter. The *white arrow* corresponds to the location of the aspiration catheter. **(f)** Post-thrombectomy DSA, right ICA injection. Note discrepancy in the size of the M2 branches, illustrating why the use of a J-shaped guidewire is preferable.

9.3 Pearls and Pitfalls

- Residual stenosis after SR thrombectomy may be a sign of underlying intracranial atherosclerosis. If the degree of residual stenosis is moderate–severe and there are no contraindications for immediate dual antiplatelet therapy, intracranial stenting could be considered (▶ Fig. 9.9). Balloon angioplasty alone may be warranted in cases with concern for hemorrhagic transformation (such as when a large ischemic core is present on noncontrast CT or CTP imaging), because although ideal, antiplatelet therapy is not mandatory in such cases.
- If severe underlying stenosis is suspected and significant resistance is encountered while attempting to withdraw the fully deployed SR, resheathing the device with a microcatheter and aborting SR thrombectomy altogether, rather than applying additional pulling force, can avoid vessel rupture and a disastrous complication. In such cases, balloon angioplasty or stenting is considered for primary treatment (Chapter 11 "Proximal MCA Occlusion—Angioplasty and Stenting").
- Local vasospasm can occur as a result of vessel irritation by the SR, especially in cases with tortuous anatomy (▶ Fig. 9.10). Local infusion of verapamil intra-arterially (5–10 mg) is effective in such cases. It can be performed through either the intermediate catheter or even the microcatheter positioned directly in the affected artery.

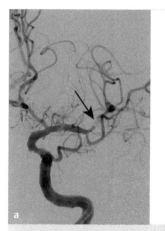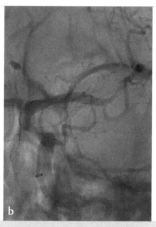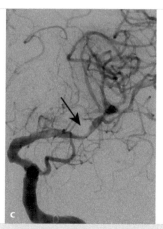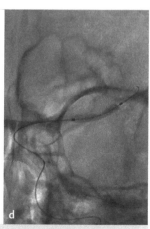

Fig. 9.9 An example of residual severe stenosis after thrombectomy treated with stent placement. **(a)** Digital subtraction angiogram (DSA), anteroposterior (AP) view, showing a clot within the proximal M2 (*arrow*). **(b)** A stent retriever (SR) (Trevo [Stryker]) is deployed, and a left internal carotid artery (ICA) injection is performed. A "temporary endovascular bypass" is achieved. **(c)** Post-thrombectomy DSA showing a suspected underlying severe residual stenosis (*arrow*). **(d)** Fluoroscopy showing deployment of a 2.25 mm × 14 mm balloon-mounted stent (Integrity [Medtronic]) to treat the underlying stenosis.

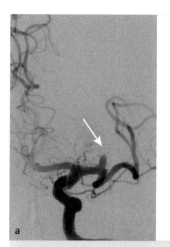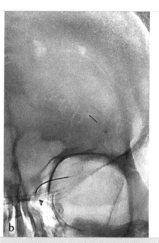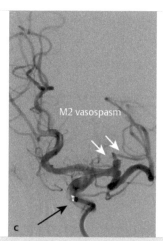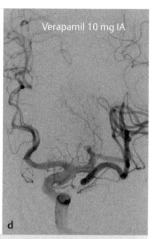

Fig. 9.10 An example of local vasospasm post-stent-retriever (post-SR) thrombectomy, treated with verapamil infusion. **(a)** Digital subtraction angiogram (DSA), anteroposterior (AP) view, left middle cerebral artery (MCA) M2 occlusion (*arrow*). Note the 90 degree M1-M2 angle. **(b)** Fluoroscopy showing the EmboTrap SR (Cerenovus). **(c)** Post-thrombectomy DSA showing vasospasm of the previously occluded M2 segment (*white arrows*). The *black arrow* points to the location of the intermediate catheter that was used to slowly infuse 10 mg of verapamil. **(d)** DSA, left internal carotid artery (ICA) injection, performed several minutes after the infusion shows a fully patent left M2 segment.

9.4 Cases with Videos and Images

9.4.1 Case 9.1 Long Sheath, Intermediate Catheter, and Stent Retriever for M1 Occlusion

A patient with sudden onset of right hemiparesis and aphasia, National Institutes of Health Stroke Scale (NIHSS) score > 20, with unknown time of symptom onset. The treatment strategy described here is one of the most common approaches we use for proximal middle cerebral artery (MCA) occlusions (▶ **Video 9.1**; ▶ Fig. 9.11, ▶ Fig. 9.12, ▶ Fig. 9.13, ▶ Fig. 9.14, ▶ Fig. 9.15, ▶ Fig. 9.16, ▶ Fig. 9.17)

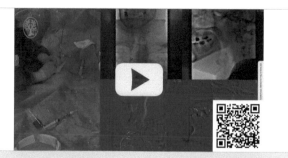

Video 9.1 Long Sheath, Intermediate Catheter, and Stent Retriever for M1 Occlusion.

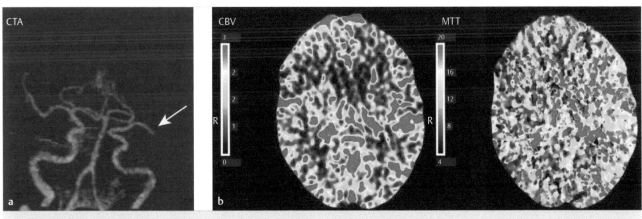

Fig. 9.11 Baseline noninvasive imaging. **(a)** Computed tomographic angiography (CTA), three-dimensional (3D) reconstruction, showing left M1 occlusion (*arrow*). **(b)** CT perfusion (CTP) images show the left hemisphere at risk: preserved cerebral blood volume (CBV; left) and prolonged mean transit time (MTT; right).

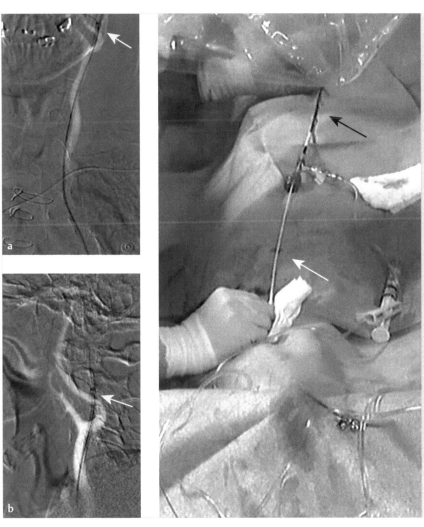

Fig. 9.12 Establishing access into the left internal carotid artery (ICA). Roadmap, **(a)** anteroposterior (AP) and **(b)** lateral views, showing delivery of the 0.088-inch inner diameter long guide sheath (*arrow*, Neuron Max, [Penumbra]) over a 0.035-inch guidewire and VTK catheter (Cook). Note straightening of the proximal cervical ICA curve, best appreciated on the lateral view. **(c)** Photograph showing the long sheath (*black arrow*) being delivered over the VTK catheter (*white arrow*).

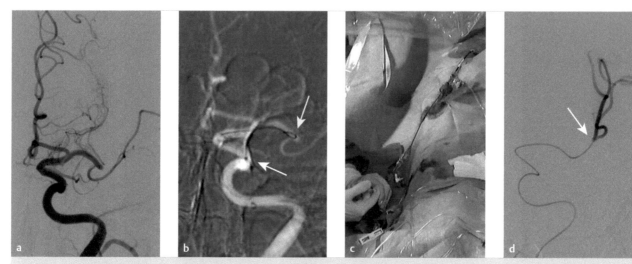

Fig. 9.13 Baseline digital subtraction angiogram (DSA) and traversing the M1 occlusion. **(a)** SA, anteroposterior (AP) view, left internal carotid artery (ICA) injection, showing distal left M1 occlusion. **(b)** Roadmap, left ICA injection, showing crossing the lesion with a "J"-shaped 0.014-inch guidewire (*yellow arrow*, Synchro [Stryker]). This allows the guidewire to remain in the largest branch. The *white arrow* points to the tip of the 0.025-inch microcatheter (Velocity [Penumbra]). The *white arrow* points to the tip of the Sofia 6F aspiration catheter (MicroVention). **(c)** Photograph, showing a superselective injection performed through the microcatheter using a 3-mL syringe. **(d)** DSA, superselective injection through the microcatheter (*arrow*). This confirms safe positioning of the microcatheter within a distal middle cerebral artery (MCA) branch. It is now safe to proceed with thrombectomy.

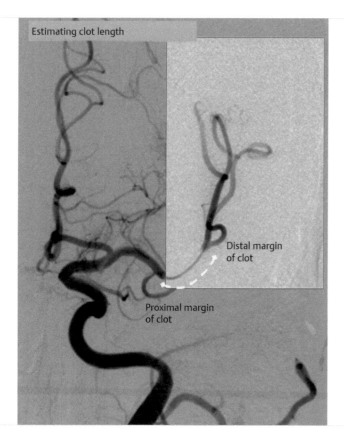

Estimating clot length

Distal margin of clot

Proximal margin of clot

Fig. 9.14 Estimating clot size on digital subtraction angiogram (DSA). DSA, anteroposterior (AP) view, showing a composite left internal carotid artery (ICA) injection and microcatheter injection (marked with the red rectangle). The *dashed yellow line* represents the filling defect caused by the clot. Estimation of the clot size helps selection of the appropriate size of stent retriever (SR) and with positioning of the SR to ensure successful thrombectomy.

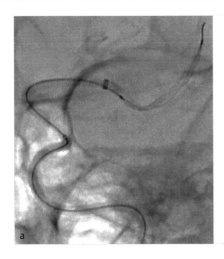
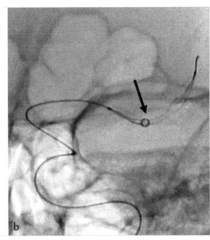

Fig. 9.15 Stent-retriever (SR) thrombectomy is performed. **(a)** Fluoroscopy, high magnification, working projection, showing deployed Tigertriever SR (Rapid Medical). The SR's braided design allows adjustment of its diameter. **(b)** Fluoroscopy, also high magnification, showing the aspiration catheter now advanced further and corking the proximal end of the clot (*arrow*).

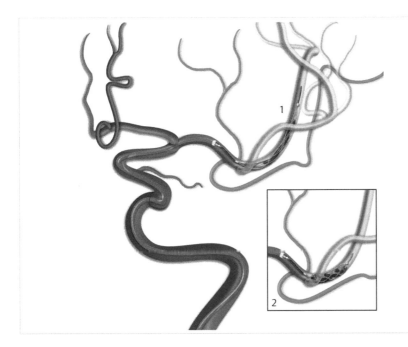

Fig. 9.16 Artist's illustration of deploying and withdrawing Tigertriever device. In step 1, the stent retriever (SR) is unsheathed. In step 2, using the adjustable handle, the operator partially compresses the length of the device, which increases its diameter and more effectively captures the clot. (© Thieme/Jennifer Pryll)

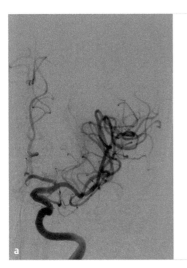
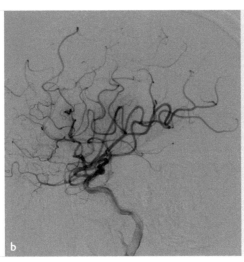

Fig. 9.17 Digital subtraction angiogram (DSA) after thrombectomy. DSA, **(a)** anteroposterior (AP) and **(b)** lateral views, showing excellent revascularization of the M1 occlusion.

9.4.2 Case 9.2 Balloon Guide Catheter, Intermediate Catheter, and Stent Retriever for M1 Occlusion

This patient had sudden onset of left hemiparesis and neglect. In this case, a balloon guide catheter (BGC) is used to add the advantage of proximal flow arrest for stent retriever (SR) plus aspiration thrombectomy (▶ Video 9.2; ▶ Fig. 9.18, ▶ Fig. 9.19, ▶ Fig. 9.20, ▶ Fig. 9.21, ▶ Fig. 9.22, ▶ Fig. 9.23).

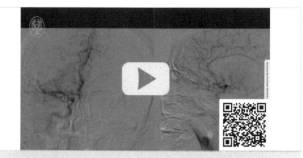

Video 9.2 Balloon Guide Catheter, Intermediate Catheter, and Stent Retriever for M1 Occlusion.

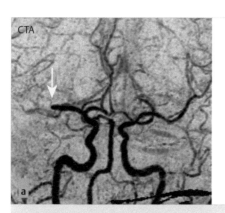
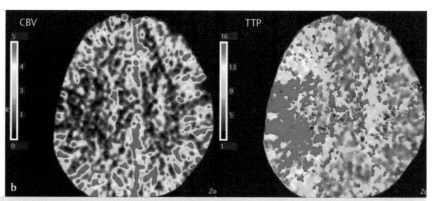

Fig. 9.18 Baseline noninvasive imaging. (a) Computed tomographic angiography (CTA), three-dimensional (3D) reconstruction, showing a distal right M1 occlusion (*arrow*). (b) CT perfusion (CTP) images show a small ischemic core but otherwise preservation of cerebral blood volume (CBV, left) and increased time-to-peak (TTP, right).

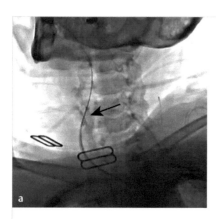
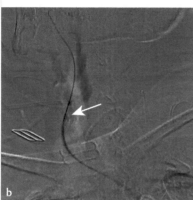
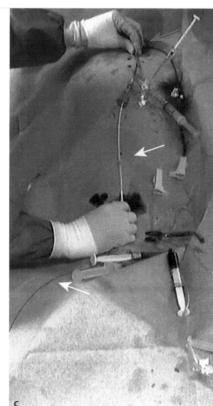

Fig. 9.19 Establishing access into the right internal carotid artery (ICA) with a balloon guide catheter (BGC). (a) Fluoroscopy and (b) roadmap, anteroposterior (AP) views, showing delivery of a BGC (Walrus, Q'Apel Medical; *arrow* in each image) over a 0.035-inch guidewire and VTK catheter (Cook). (c) Photograph, showing the BGC being delivered over the VTK catheter (*yellow arrow*) and the guidewire (*white arrow*). A 9-French (F) short sheath is required for such cases (*red arrow*).

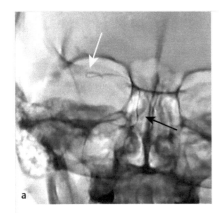

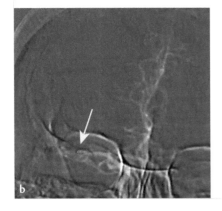

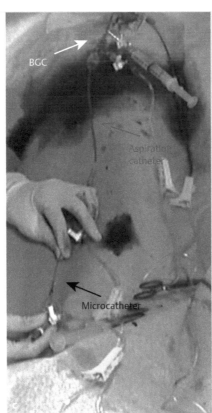

Fig. 9.20 Traversing the M1 occlusion. **(a)** Fluoroscopy and **(b)** roadmap, anteroposterior (AP) views, showing a "J"-shaped 0.014-inch guidewire (*yellow arrow*; Synchro [Stryker]) traversing the occlusion. The *black arrow* points to the tip of the 0.025-inch microcatheter (Velocity [Penumbra]). **(c)** Photograph, showing the balloon guide catheter (BGC) (*white arrow*), intermediate aspiration catheter (*red arrow*; React [Medtronic]), and microcatheter (*black arrow*).

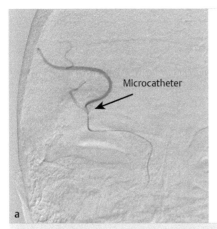

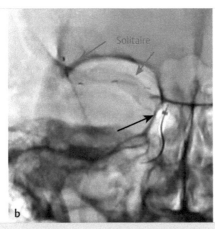

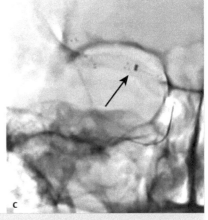

Fig. 9.21 Stent-retriever (SR) thrombectomy. **(a)** Digital subtraction angiogram (DSA), superselective injection, right middle cerebral artery (MCA), confirming good positioning of the microcatheter (*arrow*) prior to SR delivery. **(b)** Fluoroscopy, anteroposterior (AP) view, showing delivery of the SR (*red arrows*; Solitaire [Medtronic]). The *black arrow* points to the aspiration catheter. **(c)** Fluoroscopy, showing withdrawal of the SR. The aspiration catheter is advanced into the M1 (*arrow*) until the operator feels a "catch" indicating engagement of the proximal end of the clot into the catheter.

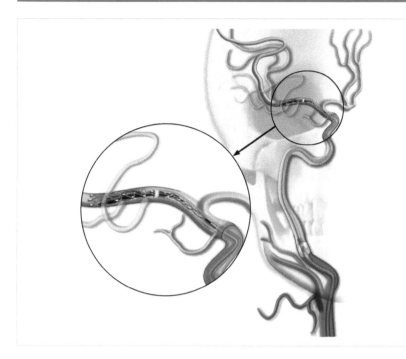

Fig. 9.22 Artist's illustration of stent-retriever (SR) thrombectomy. The balloon of the guide catheter is inflated, resulting in flow arrest through the internal carotid artery (ICA). Once the SR and clot are partially engaged into the aspiration catheter, all three are withdrawn into the guide catheter. The circled area shows higher magnification of the clot position during thrombectomy. (© Thieme/Jennifer Pryll)

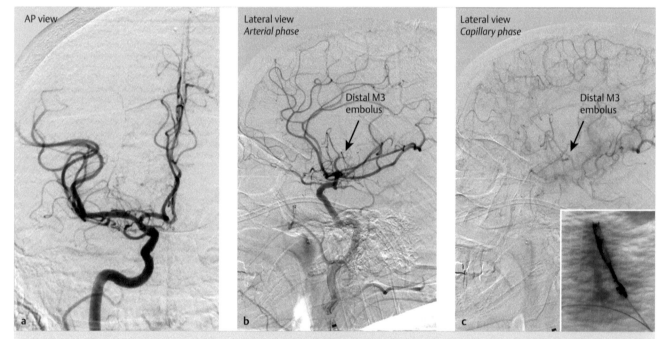

Fig. 9.23 Digital subtraction angiogram (DSA) after stent-retriever (SR) thrombectomy. **(a)** DSA, anteroposterior (AP) view, showing revascularization of the M1 occlusion. **(b)** DSA, lateral view, arterial phase, showing a distal M3 filling defect (*arrow*). **(c)** DSA, lateral view, capillary phase, confirming that distal embolization occurred in the M3 territory (*arrow*). Therefore, the final reperfusion grade is thrombolysis in cerebral infarction (TICI) grade 2C, rather than 3. Given the relatively small size of the residual perfusion deficit and its right-sided location, no further intervention was indicated. Solitaire SR capturing a thrombus removed during the case is shown in the inset photograph.

9.4.3 Case 9.3 Stent Retriever for M2 Occlusion and Vasospasm

A patient with a proximal middle cerebral artery (MCA) occlusion is treated with stent-retriever (SR) thrombectomy. Post-thrombectomy, MCA vasospasm occurred. This case illustrates intraprocedural recognition and management of vasospasm (▶ **Video 9.3**; ▶ Fig. 9.24, ▶ Fig. 9.25, ▶ Fig. 9.26, ▶ Fig. 9.27, ▶ Fig. 9.28, ▶ Fig. 9.29).

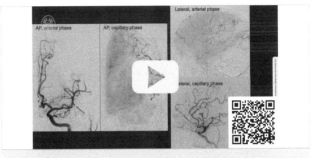

Video 9.3 Stent Retriever for M2 Occlusion and Vasospasm.

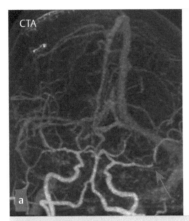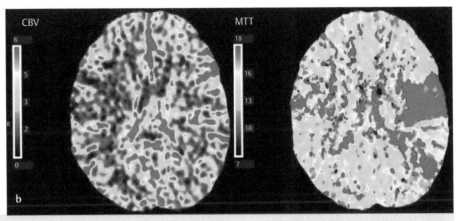

Fig. 9.24 Baseline noninvasive imaging. **(a)** Computed tomographic angiography (CTA) images demonstrating critical left M2 occlusion (*arrow*). **(b)** CT perfusion (CTP) maps show preserved cerebral blood volume (CBV; left) and increased mean transit time (MTT; right) within the left M2 territory.

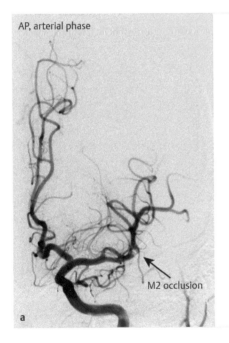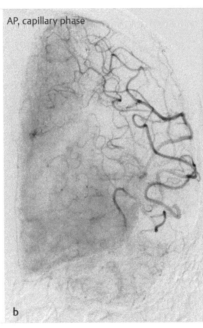

M2 occlusion

Fig. 9.25 Baseline digital subtraction angiogram (DSA). **(a)** DSA, anteroposterior (AP) view, left internal carotid artery (ICA) injection, arterial phase, showing proximal left M2 middle cerebral artery (MCA) occlusion (*arrow*). **(b)** DSA, AP view, capillary phase. The flow-limiting effect of this short occluded M2 segment is appreciated.

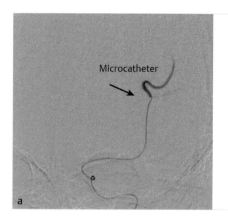

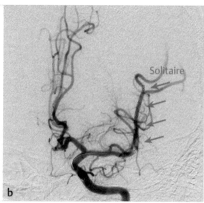

Fig. 9.26 Stent-retriever (SR) thrombectomy. **(a)** Digital subtraction angiogram (DSA), super-selective injection, left middle cerebral artery (MCA), confirming positioning of the micro-catheter within the M3 branch (*arrow*). **(b)** DSA, anteroposterior (AP) view, showing deployed Solitaire SR (*arrows*; [Medtronic]). There is now restoration of flow because the SR pushed the thrombus and partially recanalized the vessel.

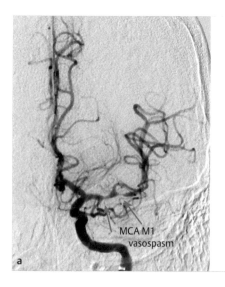

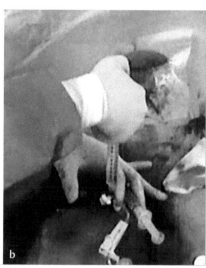

Fig. 9.27 Stent-retriever (SR) thrombectomy–induced vasospasm. **(a)** Post-thrombectomy digital subtraction angiogram (DSA), anteroposterior (AP) view, showing left middle cerebral artery (MCA) M1 vasospasm (*arrows*), likely as a result of irritation of the vessel while withdrawing the clot, SR, and aspiration catheter. This can be effectively treated by local intra-arterial infusion of a calcium channel blocker such as verapamil (10–20 mg over several minutes). **(b)** Photograph showing administration of verapamil through the guide catheter.

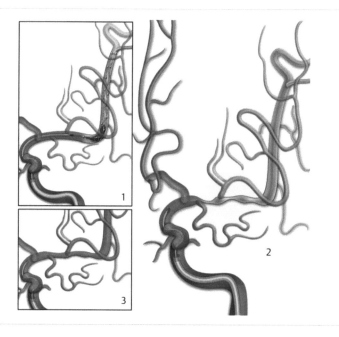

Fig. 9.28 Artist's illustration of vasospasm management after thrombectomy. In step 1, stent-retriever (SR) thrombectomy is performed. Vessel angulation such as seen in this case can predispose to spasm. Step 2 shows left M1 vasospasm causing critical residual stenosis (highlighted area). If the vasospasm is untreated, it can result in new thrombus formation. Repeat angiography postinfusion is illustrated in step 3. Improved patency of the proximal middle cerebral artery (MCA) is achieved. (© Thieme/Jennifer Pryll)

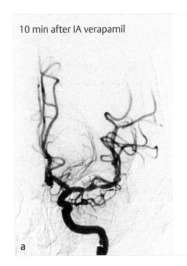

10 min after IA verapamil

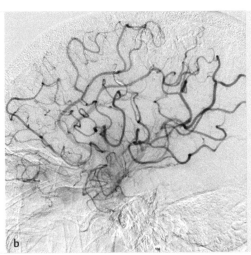

a

b

Fig. 9.29 Final digital subtraction angiogram (DSA) after thrombectomy. **(a)** DSA, anteroposterior (AP) view, showing partially improved left M1 diameter. The verapamil infusion can be repeated; however, it is often not necessary. The therapeutic effect of the verapamil will peak within 20 to 30 minutes after its infusion. **(b)** DSA, lateral view, showing fully patent left middle cerebral artery (MCA) with thrombolysis in cerebral infarction (TICI) 3 reperfusion.

9.4.4 Case 9.4 Multiple Passes with Stent Retriever and Failed Recanalization

A patient with a proximal right middle cerebral artery (MCA) occlusion is immediately taken for thrombectomy. There is a high ischemic core burden in this case, depicted on baseline noncontrast computed tomography (CT) and CT perfusion (CTP) imaging (▶ **Video 9.4**; ▶ Fig. 9.30, ▶ Fig. 9.31, ▶ Fig. 9.32, ▶ Fig. 9.33, ▶ Fig. 9.34).

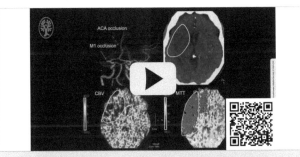

Video 9.4 Multiple Passes with Stent Retriever and Failed Recanalization.

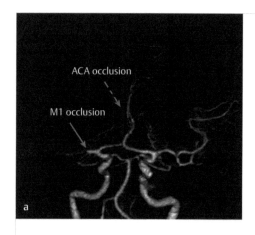
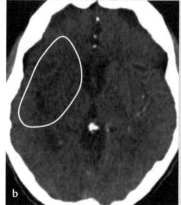
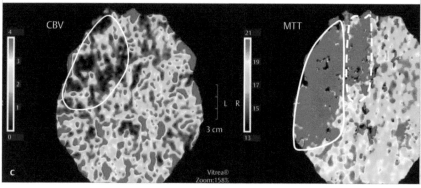

Fig. 9.30 Baseline noninvasive imaging. (a) Computed tomographic angiography (CTA), three-dimensional (3D) reconstruction, showing right M1 occlusion (arrow). There is also a right anterior cerebral artery (ACA) occlusion present (dashed arrow). (b) A large area of ischemic core (outlined area) can be appreciated on noncontrast head CT. (c) CT perfusion (CTP) images confirming a large ischemic core with reduced cerebral blood volume (CBV; left). Delayed mean transit time (MTT; right) is seen within the right middle cerebral artery (MCA) (solid line) and right ACA (broken line) territories.

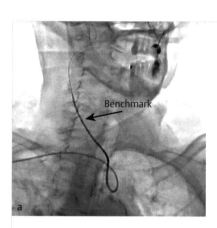
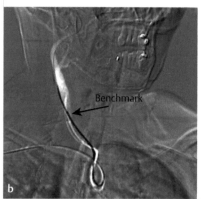
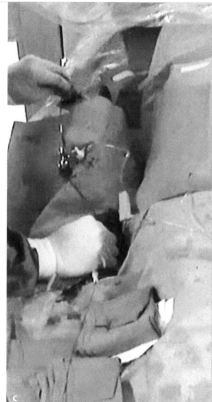

Fig. 9.31 Establishing access into the right internal carotid artery (ICA) using radial access. (a) Fluoroscopy and (b) roadmap, anteroposterior (AP) views, showing delivery of a Benchmark 0.071-inch guide catheter (arrow; Penumbra) into the right ICA. Radial access was chosen in this case because unfavorable arch anatomy was appreciated on baseline computed tomographic angiography (CTA). (c) Photograph showing the guide catheter being advanced over a 0.035-inch guidewire.

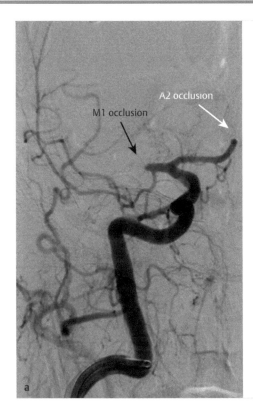

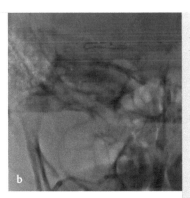

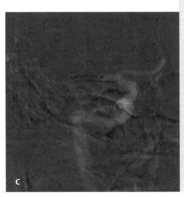

Fig. 9.32 Crossing the lesion. **(a)** Digital subtraction angiogram (DSA), anteroposterior (AP) view, right internal carotid artery (ICA) injection showing right M1 middle cerebral artery (MCA) occlusion (*black arrow*). There is also a proximal anterior cerebral artery (ACA) A2 occlusion (*white arrow*). **(b)** Fluoroscopy and **(c)** roadmap, AP view, a 0.014-inch guidewire and microcatheter are used to cross the M1 occlusion.

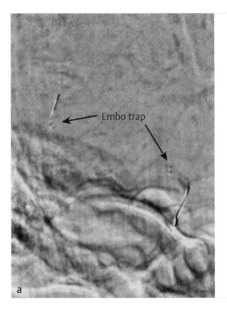

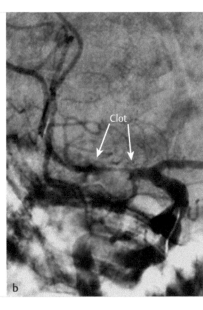

Fig. 9.33 Deploying EmboTrap stent retriever (SR). **(a)** Fluoroscopy, anteroposterior (AP) view, showing EmboTrap stent retriever (*arrows*; Cerenovus) positioned and unsheathed in the proximal right middle cerebral artery (MCA). **(b)** Digital subtraction angiogram (DSA), AP view, right internal carotid artery (ICA) injection showing a "temporary endovascular bypass." The EmboTrap pushed the clot to the side of the M1 (*arrows* correspond to the proximal and distal ends of the thrombus), thus temporarily restoring blood flow.

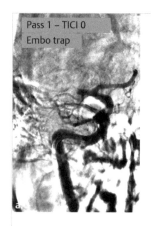

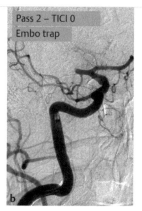

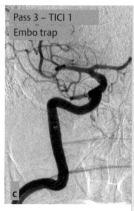

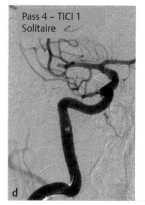

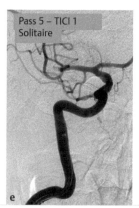

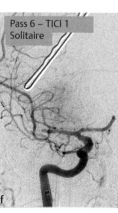

Fig. 9.34 Failed multiple rounds of stent-retriever (SR) thrombectomy. **(a–c)** Digital subtraction angiogram (DSA), anteroposterior (AP) view, right internal carotid artery (ICA) injection showing persistent proximal middle cerebral artery (MCA) occlusion despite three passes of the EmboTrap SR. **(d–f)** DSA, AP view, right ICA injection. An additional three passes of thrombectomy were performed using a Solitaire SR (Medtronic). Given the large stroke burden present on baseline imaging, the multiple thrombectomy attempts that failed to revascularize the MCA, and the increasing risk of vessel injury with three further passes, the decision was made to abort the procedure.

10 Proximal Middle Cerebral Artery Occlusion—Aspiration

General Description

Aspiration-first approach, direct aspiration, contact aspiration, and simply ADAPT (A Direct Aspiration First Pass Technique) are all common names for a versatile approach to thrombectomy for large vessel occlusion (LVO) using modern aspiration catheters. With technological advances in aspiration catheters and pumps resulting in improved trackability and aspiration power coupled with simplicity and cost-effectiveness, aspiration has become a common approach to thrombectomy.

Keywords: Aspiration, middle cerebral artery, ophthalmic artery, thrombectomy

10.1 Anatomical and Imaging Aspects

- We commonly rely on the aspiration-first approach for cases with well-organized occlusions and mild-to-moderate clot burden (▶ Fig. 10.1), reserving the use of stent retrievers (SR) for cases with massive clot burden where otherwise multiple aspiration attempts would be needed.
- Presently, there are no well-validated clinical or radiographic predictors (such as clot length, location, or imaging properties) capable of accurately identifying patients who may respond better to aspiration or SR-first approaches. Heavily calcified lesions are not ideal for aspiration, nor do they respond well to the SR approach (▶ Fig. 10.2). Angioplasty and stenting should be considered in such cases instead (Chapter 11 "Proximal Middle Cerebral Artery Occlusion—Angioplasty and Stenting").
- Significant tortuosity of the intracranial internal carotid artery (ICA) will interfere with aspiration catheter navigation toward the middle cerebral artery (MCA) occlusion, often making catheter delivery more difficult. Technical tips to overcome such anatomical challenges are discussed in the following text.

10.2 Technique and Key Steps

- Failure to deliver the aspiration catheter to the occlusion site is one of the main reasons of aspiration "failure." Reliable distal guide catheter support is critical to ensure that the aspiration catheter safely and quickly tracks (▶ Fig. 10.3). Modern 0.088-inch guide catheters with extended length (100–110 cm), softer distal segments, and rigid proximal support are ideal for this task (Ballast [Balt], TrackStar or Zoom 88 [Imperative Care]) and will accommodate most available 6-French (F) outer diameter aspiration catheters.
- Modern balloon guide catheters (BGCs), such as the Walrus (Q'Apel Medical), with a 0.087-inch inner diameter can be used to take advantage of proximal flow arrest (▶ Fig. 10.4).

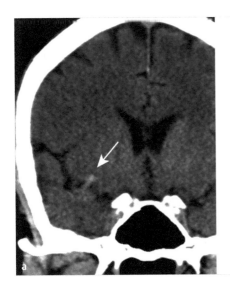
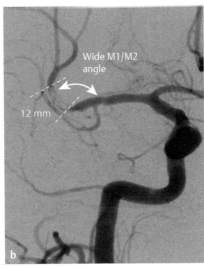

Wide M1/M2 angle

12 mm

Fig. 10.1 Example of proximal M2 occlusion suitable for aspiration thrombectomy. **(a)** Non-contrast computed tomography (CT), coronal view. There is a focal hyperdensity (*arrow*), representing a fresh clot. No underlying calcifications are seen. **(b)** Digital subtraction angiography (DSA), axial view, showing a proximal M2 occlusion. A partially occlusive clot is seen. The filling defect measures 12 mm (*yellow dashed lines*). The middle cerebral artery (MCA) angle at the proximal occlusion is wide (*curved white arrow*). Aspiration alone is likely to achieve complete recanalization in this case and is a reasonable approach to pursue.

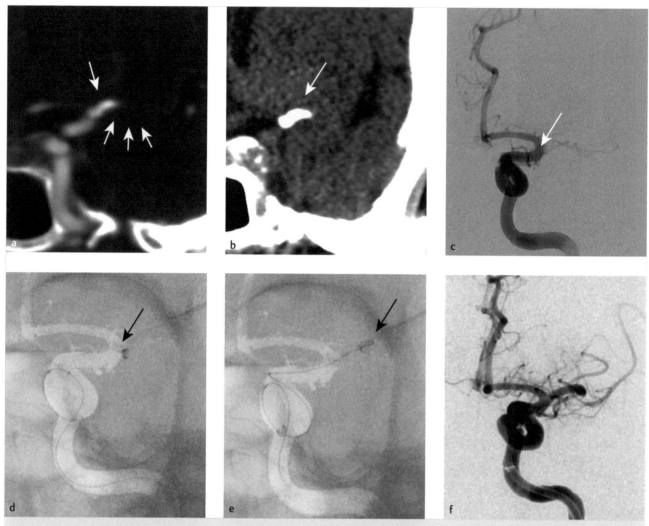

Fig. 10.2 Heavily calcified plaque resistant to aspiration thrombectomy. **(a)** Computed tomographic angiography (CTA), coronal view, showing lack of contrast opacification within the left M1 (*yellow arrows*). The *white arrow* points to a calcification. **(b)** Noncontrast computed tomography (CT), coronal view. A hyperdense lesion representing a large intracranial calcification (*arrow*) is easier to visualize on this image than on the CTA image. Unlike hyperdense clots (which normally do not exceed 50–60 Hounsfield units [HU]), these calcifications have much higher HU values above 100. **(c)** Digital subtraction angiography (DSA), axial view, confirming left M1 occlusion. Note the shadow of the embolus (calcification) protruding into the internal carotid artery (ICA) terminus (*arrow*). **(d)** DSA, roadmap, showing the tip of the aspiration catheter (*arrow*; Zoom 71 [Imperative Care]) just barely advancing into the middle cerebral artery (MCA) M1 segment. Aspiration alone is unsuccessful. **(e)** DSA, roadmap, showing attempts to cross the lesion with a 0.014-inch guidewire (*arrow*; Synchro [Stryker]), also unsuccessful. **(f)** DSA, after numerous attempts. Only thrombolysis in cerebral infarction (TICI) grade 1 reperfusion was achieved.

- Avoiding crossing the occlusion with a guidewire or microcatheter when delivering the aspiration catheter to the target location is ideal to prevent distal embolization (▶ Fig. 10.5). The "J"-shaped tip of the guidewire helps achieve extra support and avoids small perforators while navigating to the occlusion site.

- Aspiration can be performed using dedicated manufactured aspiration pumps or manual aspiration with a syringe. When no SR is used, the pump or syringe can be directly connected to the aspiration catheter (▶ Fig. 10.6), reducing the number of connecting elements (such as a three-way or rotating hemostatic valve), which can decrease aspiration power.

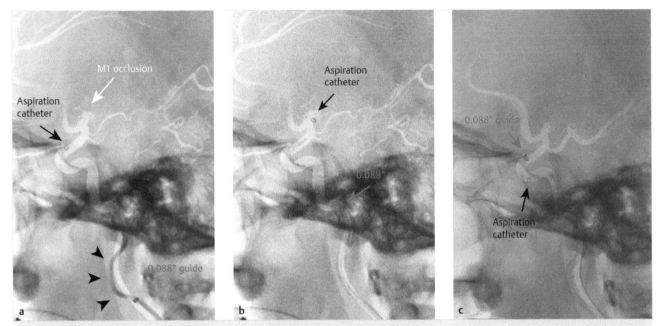

Fig. 10.3 Effect of guide catheter position on aspiration catheter trackability. **(a)** Digital subtraction angiography (DSA), roadmap, lateral view, showing a guide catheter (*red arrow*; Zoom 0.088-inch [Imperative Care]) in the proximal cervical internal carotid artery (ICA) segment. In this case of M1 occlusion (*yellow arrow*), the operator attempted to advance the aspiration catheter (6F Sofia [MicroVention]) directly without using a microcatheter or guidewire for extra support. Note how the tip of the Sofia catheter is caught on the ophthalmic artery (OA) origin (*black arrow*). Additional force applied to the aspiration catheter to push it forward only creates catheter redundancy more proximally (*arrowheads*). **(b)** DSA, roadmap, showing that by advancing the guide catheter into the petrous ICA segment (the *red arrow* points to the tip of the Zoom 0.088-inch guide catheter), another attempt of navigating the aspiration catheter leads to the catheter easily passing the OA and accessing the occlusion (*black arrow*). **(c)** DSA, roadmap showing the guide catheter advanced into the paraclinoid segment of the ICA (*red arrow*) while the aspiration catheter is pulled back under continuous aspiration (*black arrow*). This minimizes the distance the aspiration catheter travels until it reaches the guide, thus reducing the chance for losing the clot, clot breakdown, and distal embolization.

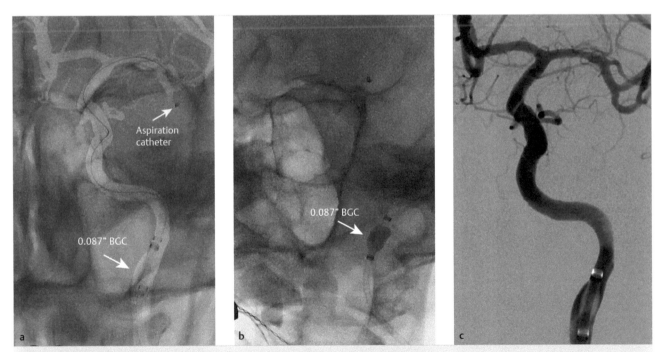

Fig. 10.4 Balloon guide catheter (BGC) and direct aspiration. **(a)** Digital subtraction angiography (DSA), roadmap, left internal carotid artery (ICA) injection, anteroposterior (AP) view, showing a 0.087-inch inner diameter BGC (*white arrow*; Walrus [Q'Apel Medical]) used to perform proximal M2 aspiration thrombectomy (*yellow arrow*; Zoom 0.071-inch [Imperative Care]). **(b)** Fluoroscopy, showing inflated BGC (*arrow*). The aspiration catheter can now be slowly withdrawn. **(c)** DSA, post-thrombectomy, showing patency of the previously occluded middle cerebral artery (MCA).

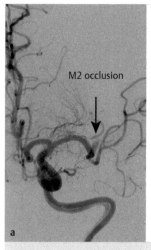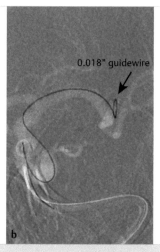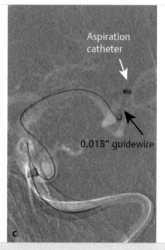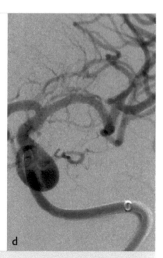

Fig. 10.5 Optimal delivery of aspiration catheter to the occlusion site. **(a)** Digital subtraction angiography (DSA), left internal carotid artery (ICA) injection, showing occlusion of the proximal dominant M2 branch (*arrow*). **(b)** DSA, roadmap, demonstrating a "J"-shaped 0.018-inch guidewire (*arrow*; Aristotle [Scientia Vascular]) parked just proximal to the occlusion. **(c)** DSA, roadmap showing a 0.071-inch aspiration catheter (*white arrow*; large-bore catheter [Cerenovus]) pushed into the proximal portion of the clot. While advancing the aspiration catheter, the guidewire is pulled back (*black arrow*). **(d)** DSA, post-thrombectomy ICA injection showing the now patent M2 and fully reperfused downstream territory.

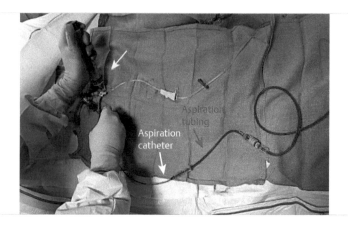

Fig. 10.6 Connecting the aspiration catheter to the pump. Photograph showing the aspiration catheter (*white arrow*; Zoom 0.071-inch [Imperative Care]) directly connected to the aspiration tubing (*red arrow*; Indigo System [Penumbra]). As the aspiration catheter is pulled back, note additional manual aspiration with a 60-mL syringe applied to the guide catheter (*yellow arrow*). This ensures capture of dislodged emboli by the guide catheter in cases of massive thrombi corked at the tip of the aspiration catheter.

10.3 Pearls and Pitfalls

- Modern aspiration catheters have excellent trackability and can be rapidly delivered all the way to the target occlusion without the use of guidewire or microcatheter support. This approach is sometimes referred to as "snaking" the catheter (▶ Fig. 10.7). Connecting the aspiration catheter to a syringe and torquing the catheter could help with navigation of the catheter through even the most tortuous anatomy (▶ Fig. 10.7).

- The origin of the ophthalmic artery (OA) is a common location for the aspiration catheter to become caught during delivery. Using a more supporting guidewire or a microcatheter with a larger diameter to reduce the catheter step-off discrepancy (▶ Fig. 10.8) is the most common maneuvers used to overcome this challenging anatomical region for aspiration. Adding a second guidewire for extra support (▶ Fig. 10.9) or using catheters specifically designed to improve aspiration catheter navigability around the OA and MCA–anterior cerebral artery (ACA) bifurcations, such as

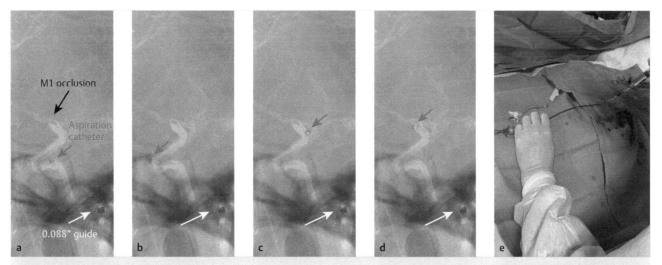

Fig. 10.7 The snake technique. **(a–d)** Digital subtraction angiography (DSA), roadmap, consecutive lateral views, showing the aspiration catheter (*red arrows* in **(a–d)**; Zoom 0.071-inch [Imperative Care]) gradually advanced into the following vessel segments: horizontal cavernous **(a)**, ophthalmic **(b)**, internal carotid artery (ICA) terminus **(c)**, and finally the M1 **(d)**. The *black arrow* in **(a)** indicates the location of the M1 occlusion prior to thrombectomy. The *yellow arrows* in **(a–d)** point to the location of the 0.088-inch guide catheter (TracStar [Imperative Care]). **(e)** Photograph showing the operator advancing and carefully torquing the aspiration catheter to improve catheter navigation through vessel tortuosity.

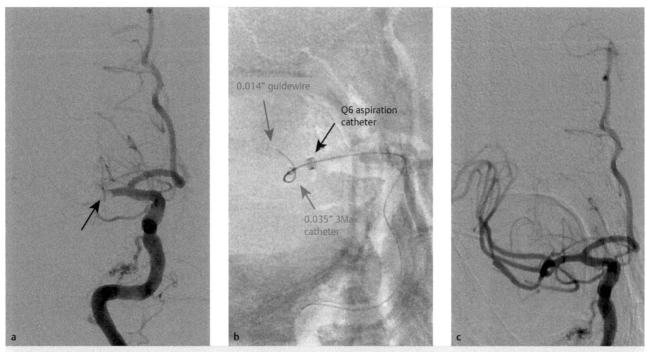

Fig. 10.8 Using a large outer diameter microcatheter for aspiration catheter delivery. **(a)** Digital subtraction angiography (DSA), anteroposterior (AP) view, showing right M1 occlusion (*black arrow*). Initially, the operator attempted to deliver the aspiration catheter (Q6 distal access catheter [MIVI]) over a 0.025-inch microcatheter (Velocity [Penumbra]) and 0.014-inch guidewire (Synchro [Stryker]), which was unsuccessful (not shown). **(b)** DSA roadmap showing the Q6 aspiration catheter (*black arrow*) successfully advanced into the occluded M1 segment. This was achieved by switching to a large outer diameter 0.035-inch catheter (*red arrow*; 3Max [Penumbra]). The *blue line* points to the 0.014-inch Synchro [Stryker] guidewire. **(c)** DSA, AP view. Patent right middle cerebral artery (MCA) trifurcation after thrombectomy.

the Wedge microcatheter (MicroVention) (▶ Fig. 10.10), is an additional trick to help with navigation of the aspiration catheter to its intracranial target.

- Although some groups propose to begin aspiration when the catheter tip is positioned proximal to the clot, we argue against such an approach. High negative aspiration forces generated by large-bore catheters and powerful pumps may

cause vessel collapse when the catheter tip is not in direct contact with the clot. Instead, we advocate partial wedging of the catheter into the clot before attempting aspiration.

- Residual thrombus within the MCA seen angiographically postaspiration, even if non-flow limiting, may result in reocclusion and therefore should be treated (▶ Fig. 10.11). If aspiration alone is not effective, we switch to an SR.

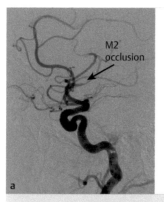 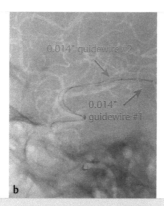 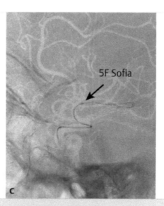 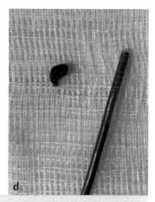

Fig. 10.9 Using a second guidewire to improve aspiration catheter trackability. **(a)** Digital subtraction angiography (DSA), lateral view, showing a proximal middle cerebral artery (MCA) M2 occlusion (*arrow*). Initial attempts to deliver the 5F Sofia aspiration catheter [MicroVention] to the occluded M2 were unsuccessful (not shown). **(b)** DSA, roadmap, showing a second 0.014-inch guidewire (*blue arrow*; Synchro [Stryker]) in parallel with the first 0.014-inch Synchro guidewire (*red arrow*). **(c)** DSA, roadmap, showing successful delivery of the aspiration catheter (*arrow*). **(d)** Photograph showing a thrombus extracted with aspiration.

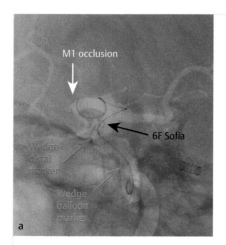 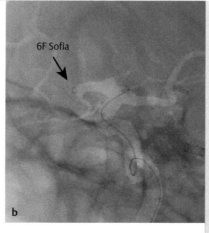

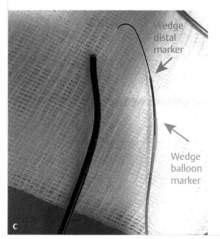 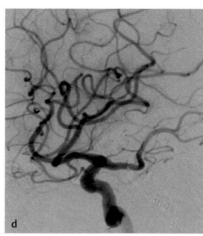

Fig. 10.10 Wedge microcatheter use. **(a)** Digital subtraction angiography (DSA), roadmap, M1 occlusion (*white arrow*). The tip of a 0.070-inch aspiration catheter (*black arrow*; 6F Sofia [MicroVention]) is caught at the ophthalmic artery (OA) origin, and additional pressure applied to the catheter is futile. The Wedge microcatheter (MicroVention) is delivered through the aspiration catheter. This microcatheter has a balloon-like larger diameter segment (0.068-inch bulb maximum diameter) starting at its proximal radiopaque marker (*blue arrow*). The distal marker corresponds to the tip of the microcatheter (*red arrow*). **(b)** DSA, road map, showing the aspiration catheter (*black arrow*) successfully navigated to the occlusion. **(c)** Photograph showing 0.072-inch aspiration catheter (Jet 7 [Penumbra]) and Wedge microcatheter. The *blue* and *red arrows* point to the proximal and distal radiopaque markers of the Wedge microcatheter. The microcatheter is compatible with 0.014- to 0.018-inch guidewires. **(d)** DSA, postaspiration thrombectomy, showing excellent angiographic outcome of the procedure.

10.4 Cases with Videos and Images

10.4.1 Case 10.1 Direct Aspiration with First-Pass Effect

In this case of an acute stroke from a middle cerebral artery (MCA) M1 occlusion, a variety of thrombectomy tools could be used first-line. The operator here chose to use a MIVI catheter, which has some unique technical nuances (▶ **Video 10.1**; ▶ Fig. 10.12, ▶ Fig. 10.13, ▶ Fig. 10.14, ▶ Fig. 10.15).

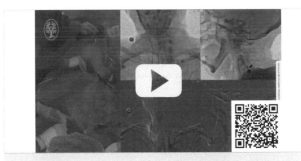

Video 10.1 Direct Aspiration with First-Pass Effect.

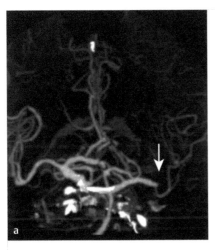

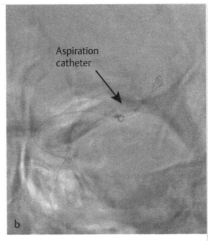

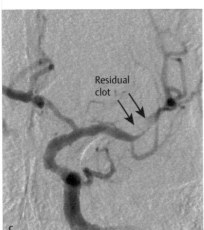

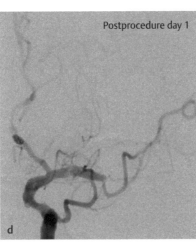

Fig. 10.11 Early reocclusion due to residual thrombus. **(a)** Computed tomographic angiography (CTA), 3D reconstruction, showing left middle cerebral artery (MCA) M1 occlusion (*arrow*). **(b)** Roadmap showing access to the occlusion site with an aspiration catheter (*arrow*). **(c)** Digital subtraction angiography (DSA), post-thrombectomy, showing restored filling distally. Although thrombolysis in cerebral infarction (TICI) 2b reperfusion was achieved, there was significant residual thrombus noted (*arrows*). No further thrombectomy attempts were performed. **(d)** DSA, anteroposterior (AP) view, showing left MCA M1 reocclusion. This study was repeated the day after aspiration thrombectomy when the patient developed acute worsening of right hemiparesis and aphasia. Stent-retriever (SR) thrombectomy was performed followed by intracranial stenting.

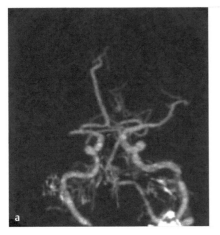

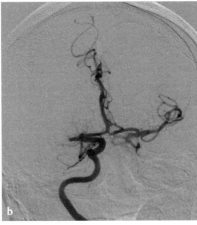

Fig. 10.12 Baseline imaging. **(a)** Computed tomographic angiography (CTA), 3D reconstruction, showing right M1 occlusion. **(b)** Digital subtraction angiography (DSA), anteroposterior (AP) view, right internal carotid artery (ICA) injection, confirming right M1 occlusion.

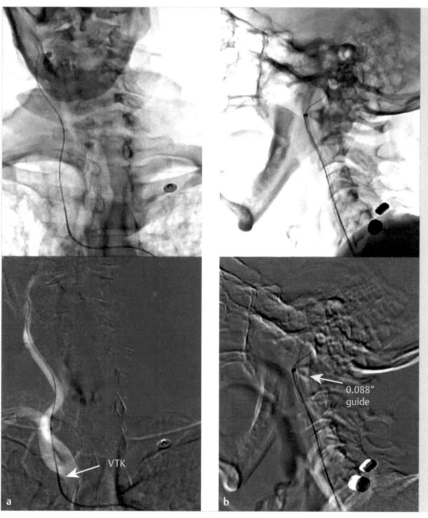

Fig. 10.13 Establishing access into the right internal carotid artery (ICA). **(a)** Fluoroscopy (top image) and roadmap (bottom image), anteroposterior (AP) views, brachiocephalic artery injection, showing catheterization of the right ICA with a 0.035-inch guidewire. A VTK catheter (*arrow*; Cook) is used to help direct the guidewire into the right carotid artery. **(b)** Fluoroscopy (top image) and roadmap (bottom image), AP views, demonstrating delivery of a 0.088-inch guidewire (*arrow*; NeuronMax [Penumbra]) into the distal right cervical ICA segment.

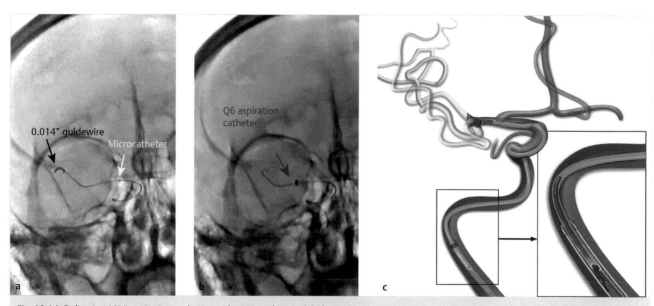

Fig. 10.14 Delivering MIVI aspiration catheter to the M1 occlusion. **(a)** Fluoroscopy, anteroposterior (AP) view. A 0.014-inch guidewire (*black arrow*; Synchro [Stryker]) and microcatheter (*yellow arrow*; Velocity [Penumbra]) are used to guide the aspiration catheter toward the M1 occlusion. **(b)** Fluoroscopy, AP view. A Q6 aspiration catheter (*blue arrow*; MIVI Neuroscience) is brought to the occlusion. **(c)** Artist's illustration of the MIVI catheter concept. The MIVI catheter is a telescopic extension of the guide catheter, allowing maximal aspiration in comparison to that for a standard aspiration catheter. High-magnification inset illustrates that the clot transitions from the MIVI catheter into the guide catheter. (**c:** © Thieme/Jennifer Pryll)

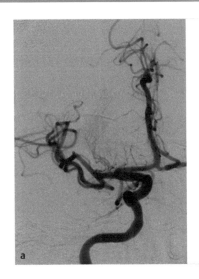
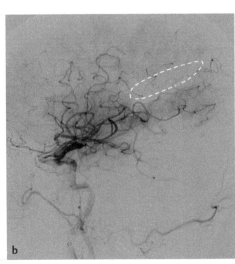

Fig. 10.15 Digital subtraction angiography (DSA) after thrombectomy. DSA, **(a)** anteroposterior (AP) and **(b)** lateral views, showing excellent revascularization of the M1 occlusion with thrombolysis in cerebral infarction (TICI) 2c reperfusion. A small distal parietal area of hypoperfusion is indicated by the *dashed region*.

10.4.2 Case 10.2 Direct Aspiration of M1 Followed by Stent Retriever for a More Distal Occlusion

The patient presented within 6 hours of stroke onset. The case illustrates how aspiration-first was used to treat an M1 occlusion followed by the use of a stent retriever (SR) for a more distal lesion (▶ **Video 10.2**; ▶ Fig. 10.16, ▶ Fig. 10.17, ▶ Fig. 10.18, ▶ Fig. 10.19).

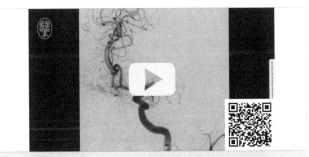

Video 10.2 Direct Aspiration of M1 Followed by Stent Retriever for a More Distal Occlusion.

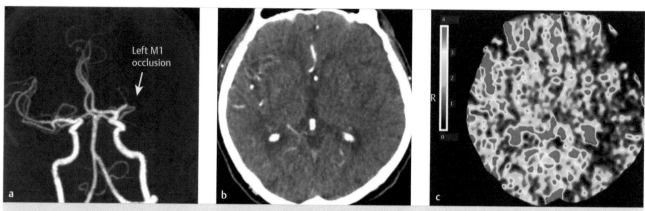

Fig. 10.16 Baseline noninvasive imaging. **(a)** Computed tomographic angiography (CTA), 3D reconstruction, showing left M1 occlusion (*arrow*). **(b)** CTA, axial view. Note poor left middle cerebral artery (MCA) territory collaterals in comparison to the right side. However, there is no obvious hypodensity and the Alberta Stroke Program Early CT Score (ASPECTS) is above 6. **(c)** CT perfusion (CTP), cerebral blood volume (CBV) showing a large core. This illustrates an infrequent scenario when perfusion imaging may incorrectly overestimate the true extent of ischemic injury. Thrombectomy is indicated in this case.

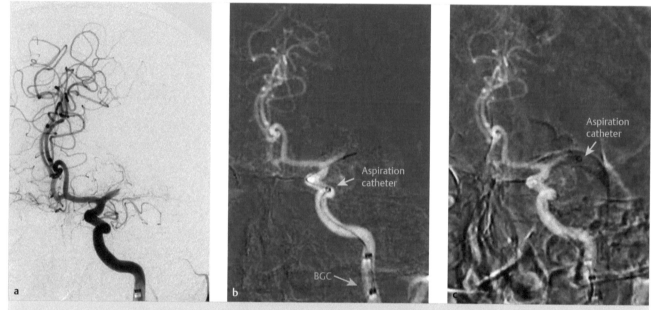

Fig. 10.17 M1 aspiration thrombectomy. **(a)** Digital subtraction angiography (DSA), anteroposterior (AP) view, left internal carotid artery (ICA) injection, showing left M1 occlusion. **(b)** Fluoroscopy, AP view, showing delivery of a 0.070-inch aspiration catheter (*green arrow*; 6F Sofia [MicroVention]). A balloon guide catheter (BGC) is used for access (*blue arrow*; Walrus [Q'Apel Medical]). **(c)** Fluoroscopy, showing the aspiration catheter at the occlusion site (*arrow*). The BGC balloon is now inflated, and aspiration thrombectomy is performed.

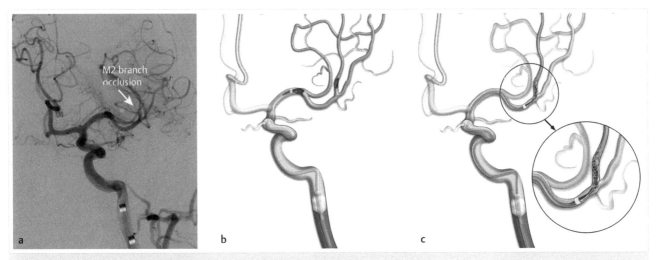

Fig. 10.18 Distal emboli with M2 occlusion. **(a)** Digital subtraction angiography (DSA), anteroposterior (AP) view, showing revascularization of the M1 occlusion. Despite using a balloon guide catheter (BGC) for flow arrest, an M2 branch occlusion can be seen, indicative of a sizable distal M2 clot (*arrow*). Further thrombectomy is indicated. The operator chose to use a stent retriever (SR). **(b)** Artist's illustration of a distal embolus breaking from the original M1 clot during aspiration thrombectomy. **(c)** Artist's illustration of performing SR thrombectomy of an M2 occlusion. The same aspiration catheter is now used to deliver a microcatheter and SR device. The inset is a magnified view of the clot captured by the SR distally and by the aspiration catheter proximally. **(b, c:** © Thieme/Jennifer Pryll)

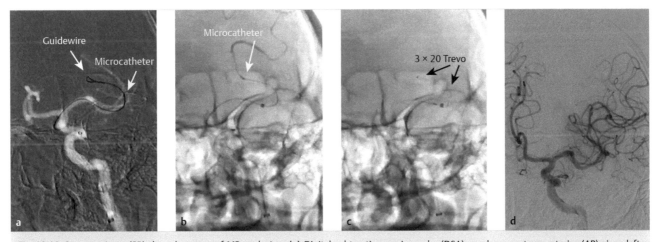

Fig. 10.19 Stent-retriever (SR) thrombectomy of M2 occlusion. **(a)** Digital subtraction angiography (DSA), roadmap, anteroposterior (AP) view, left internal carotid artery (ICA) injection, showing crossing the M2 occlusion with a guidewire (*white arrow*; Synchro [Stryker]) and a 0.021-inch Trevo Pro microcatheter (*yellow arrow*; Stryker). **(b)** Superselective injection, left middle cerebral artery (MCA), unsubtracted view, confirming good positioning of the microcatheter (*arrow*) prior to SR delivery. **(c)** Fluoroscopy showing unsheathing of the 3 × 20-mm Trevo SR (*black arrows*; Stryker). **(d)** DSA, final run, showing successful recanalization.

10.4.3 Case 10.3 Aborted Stent-Retriever Attempt and Successful Aspiration Instead

In this case of a proximal middle cerebral artery (MCA) occlusion, aspiration is performed as a rescue treatment after attempted unsuccessful primary stent-retriever (SR) thrombectomy (▶ **Video 10.3**; ▶ Fig. 10.20, ▶ Fig. 10.21, ▶ Fig. 10.22, ▶ Fig. 10.23).

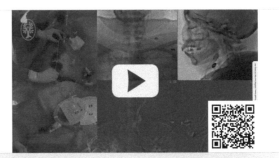

Video 10.3 Aborted Stent-Retriever Attempt and Successful Aspiration Instead.

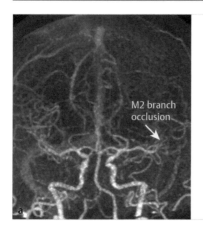

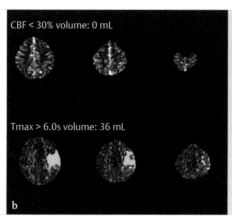

CBF < 30% volume: 0 mL

Tmax > 6.0s volume: 36 mL

Fig. 10.20 Baseline noninvasive imaging. **(a)** Computed tomographic angiography (CTA) images demonstrate left M2 occlusion (*arrow*). It is not easy to visualize the occlusion. Perfusion imaging helped alert the stroke team about the presence of large vessel occlusion (LVO) in this case. **(b)** CT perfusion (CTP) maps show preserved cerebral blood volume (CBV) < 30% (top images) and increased Tmax > 6 s (bottom images), corresponding to M2 territory branch occlusion.

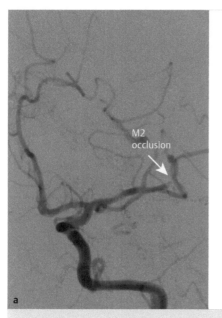

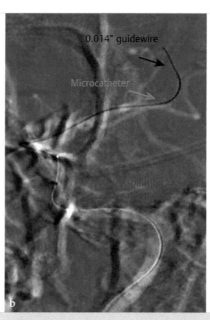

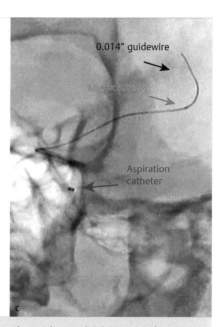

Fig. 10.21 Attempted stent-retriever (SR) thrombectomy. **(a)** SA, anteroposterior (AP) view, left internal carotid artery (ICA) injection, showing proximal left M2 middle cerebral artery (MCA) occlusion (*arrow*). **(b)** Roadmap and **(c)** fluoroscopy, AP view, showing a 0.014-inch guidewire successfully traversing the lesion (*black arrow*; Synchro [Stryker]). However, the 0.025-inch microcatheter used in this case (*blue arrow*; Velocity [Penumbra]) cannot be advanced beyond the occlusion for SR delivery. Note the location of the aspiration catheter (*green arrow*; 6F Sofia [MicroVention]) in the petrous ICA segment.

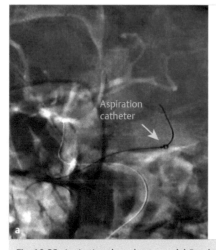

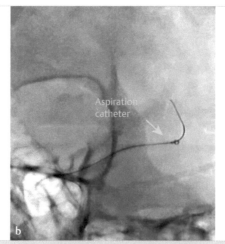

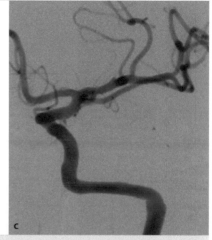

Fig. 10.22 Aspiration thrombectomy. **(a)** Roadmap and **(b)** fluoroscopy, anteroposterior (AP) view, showing that the aspiration catheter (*arrow* in each image; 6F Sofia [MicroVention]) is now advanced over the guidewire and microcatheter to the M2 occlusion for thrombectomy. **(c)** Digital subtraction angiography (DSA), final post-thrombectomy left internal carotid artery (ICA) injection, confirming successful recanalization.

10.4.4 Case 10.4 Aspiration Catheter Catches on Ophthalmic Artery; Stent Retriever is Used

This case illustrates a common scenario during aspiration thrombectomy when difficulty navigating the catheter around the paraclinoid internal carotid artery (ICA) segment is encountered (▶ Video 10.4; ▶ Fig. 10.24, ▶ Fig. 10.25, ▶ Fig. 10.26).

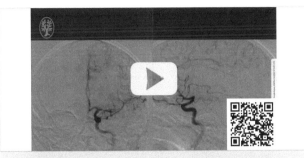

Video 10.4 Aspiration Catheter Catches on Ophthalmic Artery; Stent Retriever is Used.

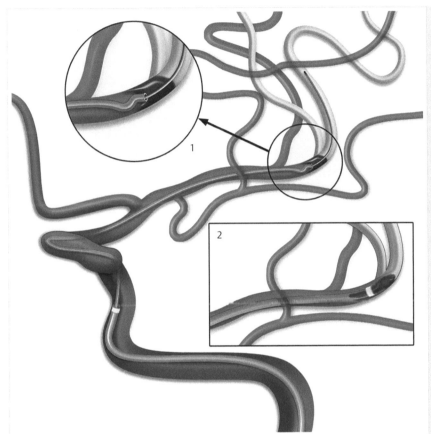

Fig. 10.23 Artist's illustration of rescue aspiration thrombectomy. In Step 1, the operator is unable to push the microcatheter across the clot despite the distal purchase from the guidewire. The inset shows the tip of the microcatheter encountering extensive resistance (*yellow* highlighted area) at the proximal end of the clot. Planned stent-retriever (SR) thrombectomy is aborted. In Step 2, aspiration comes to the rescue. (© Thieme/ Jennifer Pryll)

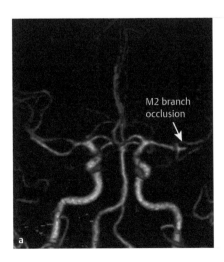

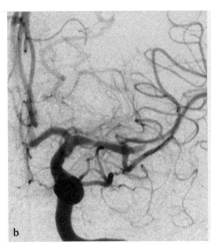

Fig. 10.24 Baseline imaging. **(a)** Computed tomographic angiography (CTA), 3D reconstruction, showing left M2 occlusion (*arrow*). **(b)** Digital subtraction angiography (DSA), left internal carotid artery (ICA) injection, anteroposterior (AP) view, demonstrating in more details that in this patient with middle cerebral artery (MCA) trifurcation occlusion, the occluded branch is the dominant one.

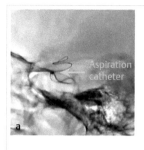
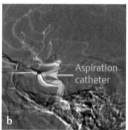
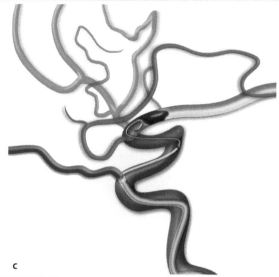

Fig. 10.25 Delivery of aspiration catheter around the cavernous segment. (a) Fluoroscopy and (b) roadmap, lateral views, showing the tip of the aspiration catheter (*arrow* in each image; 6F Sofia [MicroVention]) caught on the ophthalmic artery (OA). (c) Artist's illustration of an aspiration catheter getting stuck on the ophthalmic segment of the internal carotid artery (ICA) (highlighted by the *yellow region*). (c: © Thieme/Jennifer Pryll)

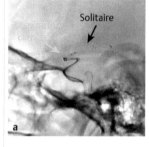
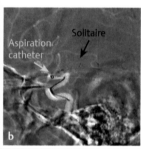
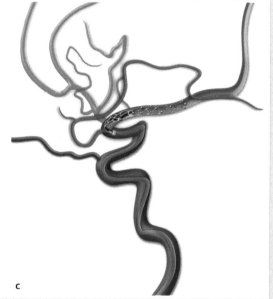

Fig. 10.26 The stent-retriever (SR) anchor technique. (a) Fluoroscopy and (b) roadmap, lateral views. The Solitaire SR (*black arrow*; Medtronic) is deployed in the middle cerebral artery (MCA). The aspiration catheter (*green arrow*; 6F Sofia [MicroVention]) can now easily track intracranially. (c) Artist's illustration of using an SR as an anchor to maneuver the aspiration catheter across the catch point of the ophthalmic artery (OA). (c: © Thieme/Jennifer Pryll)

10.4.5 Case 10.5 Direct Aspiration with Reocclusion, Underlying Atherosclerosis, and Rescue Intracranial Stenting

This case illustrates thrombectomy in a patient with underlying atherosclerosis. Aspiration alone is often unsuccessful, requiring subsequent angioplasty or stenting of such lesions (▶ **Video 10.5**; ▶ Fig. 10.27, ▶ Fig. 10.28, ▶ Fig. 10.29, ▶ Fig. 10.30, ▶ Fig. 10.31).

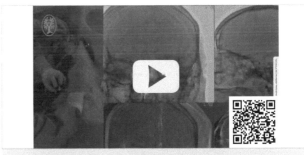

Video 10.5 Direct Aspiration with Reocclusion, Underlying Atherosclerosis, and Rescue Intracranial Stenting.

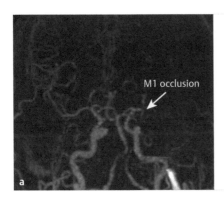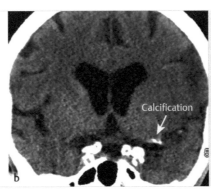

Fig. 10.27 Baseline noninvasive imaging. (a) Computed tomographic angiography (CTA), 3D reconstruction, showing left M1 occlusion (*arrow*). (b) Noncontrast computed tomography (CT), axial view, demonstrating a dense hyperdensity (*arrow*). This indicates an underlying calcification, raising suspicions for an atherosclerotic etiology of the lesion.

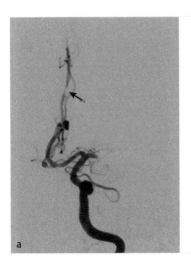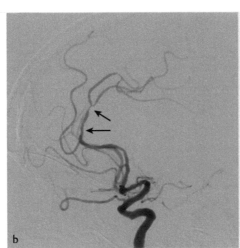

Fig. 10.28 Baseline digital subtraction angiography (DSA). DSA, (a) anteroposterior (AP) and (b) lateral views, left internal carotid artery (ICA) injection, confirming left M1 occlusion. Note diffuse intracranial atherosclerosis (*arrows*), further confirming the suspicion of underlying atherosclerotic etiology of the M1 occlusion in this case.

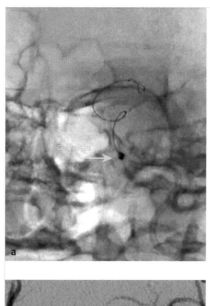

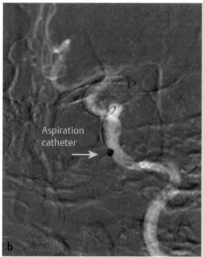

Fig. 10.29 Aspiration thrombectomy. (a) Fluoroscopy and (b) roadmap, anteroposterior (AP) view, left internal carotid artery (ICA) injection, showing delivery of a 0.070-inch aspiration catheter (*arrow* in each image; 6F Sofia [MicroVention]). (c) Digital subtraction angiography (DSA), anteroposterior (AP) view, post-thrombectomy. Severe residual M1 stenosis can be seen (*arrow*). If left untreated, middle cerebral artery (MCA) reocclusion is likely to occur. (d) Repeat DSA several minutes later showing expected reocclusion.

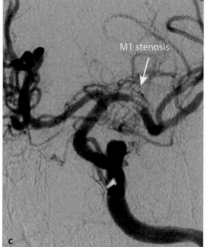

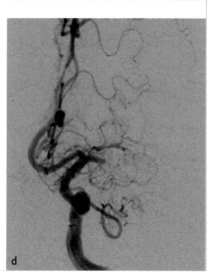

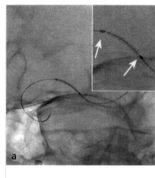

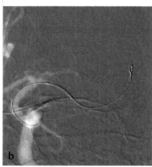

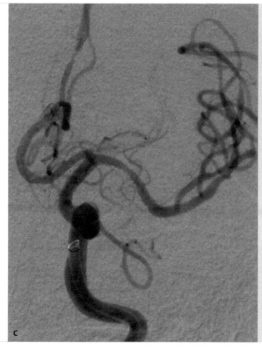

Fig. 10.30 Middle cerebral artery (MCA) stenting. (a) Fluoroscopy and (b) roadmap, anteroposterior (AP) view, showing delivery of Resolute Onyx balloon-mounted stent (Medtronic). Two radiopaque balloon markers (*arrows*) are shown in the high magnification inset. (b) Fluoroscopy, also high magnification, showing balloon inflation. (c) Digital subtraction angiography (DSA), final post-thrombectomy left internal carotid artery (ICA) injection, demonstrating patent left M1.

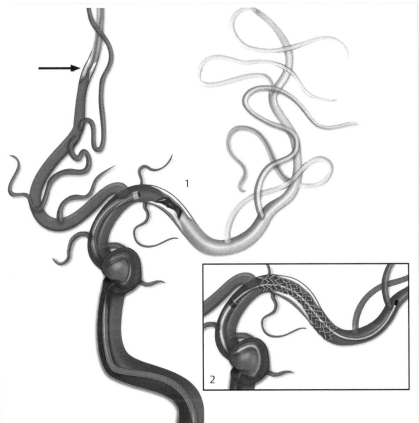

Fig. 10.31 Artist's illustration of rescue stenting. Paying attention to angiographic appearance of other vessels helps the neurointerventionists to recognize underlying atherosclerosis (*arrow*). Aspiration can be used to remove the thrombus (step 1). Rescue angioplasty or primary stenting is needed to definitively treat the lesion if severe underlying stenosis is present following aspiration thrombectomy (step 2). (© Thieme/Jennifer Pryll)

11 Proximal Middle Cerebral Artery Occlusion—Angioplasty and Stenting

General Description

The proximal middle cerebral artery (MCA) is a common location for intracranial stenosis. Intracranial stenting for acute stroke can be used as a primary approach when atherosclerosis is suspected as the underlying etiology of large vessel occlusion (LVO). Alternatively, stenting may be used as a rescue technique when angioplasty alone is not effective in maintaining sufficient patency of the affected artery or when traditional mechanical thrombectomy approaches (aspiration or stent-retriever [SR] thrombectomy) have failed to establish adequate recanalization.

Keywords: Angioplasty, atherosclerosis, balloon-mounted stent, fractional flow reserve, middle cerebral artery

11.1 Anatomical and Imaging Aspects

- Recognizing underlying atherosclerosis *prior to* performing thrombectomy can be a challenging task in a case of an MCA occlusion. Dense calcifications on noncontrast computed tomography (CT) should warn the interventionist about this potential etiology of the LVO (▶ Fig. 11.1).
- Intraprocedurally, post-thrombectomy rapid reocclusion of the affected vessel or residual stenosis following "debulking" of the clot with an aspiration catheter or SR suggests the presence of an underlying stenosis (▶ Fig. 11.2).

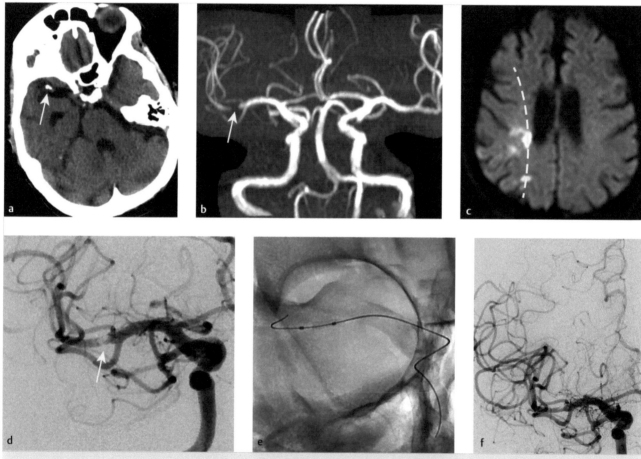

Fig. 11.1 An example of right middle cerebral artery (MCA) stenosis with a heavily calcified plaque. **(a)** Noncontrast head computed tomography (CT), axial view, showing a focal highly hyperdense region corresponding to the location of the right MCA M1 segment (*arrow*). Such heavily calcified plaque is best treated with angioplasty or stenting. **(b)** Magnetic resonance angiogram (MRA), coronal view showing a corresponding filling defect (*arrow*). The MRA alone has limited diagnostic value in this case, because it cannot be used to reliably differentiate between a short thrombus and an atherosclerotic plaque. **(c)** Magnetic resonance imaging (MRI) of the brain, diffusion-weighted sequence, with acute infarcts that partially follow the watershed MCA–anterior cerebral artery territory (*dashed line*). **(d)** Digital subtraction angiogram (DSA), anteroposterior (AP) view, right internal carotid artery (ICA) injection, showing right MCA trifurcation. The dominant M2 origin near-occlusion is seen (*arrow*). **(e)** Fluoroscopy, AP view, demonstrating balloon angioplasty with a 2.25-mm × 8-mm Trek coronary balloon (Abbott). **(f)** DSA, AP view, postintervention, showing improved patency of the affected M2 branch.

- Intracranial atherosclerosis is frequently a multifocal disease; thus, the angiographic appearance of other vessels indicating an underlying atherosclerosis helps establish the etiology and guide the operator in choosing the safest and most effective treatment approach.

11.2 Technique and Key Steps

- The two main types of stents used for intracranial stenting are self-expandable and balloon-mounted stents. An example

of a self-expandable design is the Wingspan stent (Stryker) (▶ Fig. 11.3). Predilatation (balloon angioplasty) and device exchange are required for successful stent deployment to allow for full expansion of the device.
- Balloon-mounted stents (▶ Fig. 11.2) have an advantage of simultaneous angioplasty and stent placement. However, compared with self-expandable stents, balloon-mounted stents have limited trackability characteristics when advancing the unfolded stent to the lesion prior to deployment.

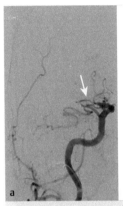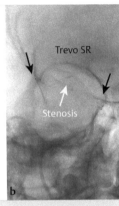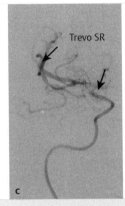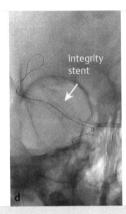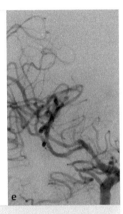

Fig. 11.2 Failed stent-retriever (SR) thrombectomy and rescue stenting. **(a)** Digital subtraction angiogram (DSA), anteroposterior (AP) view, showing right middle cerebral artery (MCA) occlusion (*arrow*). **(b)** Fluoroscopy, AP view, showing a 4-mm × 20-mm Trevo SR (Stryker) unsheathed in the affected MCA. The *black arrows* point to the proximal and distal ends of the device. Note severe constriction at the midportion of the device, indicating underlying stenosis (*yellow arrow*). **(c)** DSA, AP view, right internal carotid artery (ICA) injection with the Trevo SR in the right MCA. Minimal flow of contrast material is seen. The *black arrows* correspond to the position of the device. **(d)** Fluoroscopy, AP view, showing deployed bare metal balloon-mounted Integrity stent (*yellow arrow*; Medtronic), corresponding to the suspected location of underlying stenosis seen on previous images. **(e)** DSA, AP view, confirming restoration of blood flow post stenting.

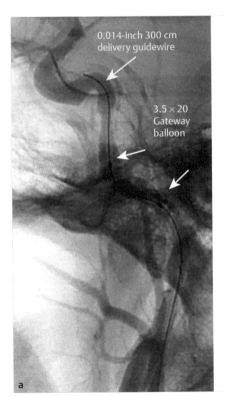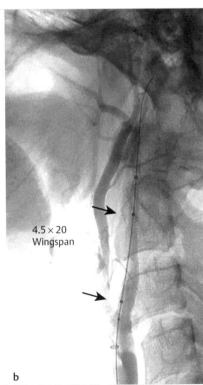

Fig. 11.3 Gateway angioplasty balloon and Wingspan stent system. **(a)** Fluoroscopy, lateral view, showing delivery of a 3.5-mm × 20-mm Gateway angioplasty balloon (Stryker). This is an over-the-wire balloon and requires a 0.014-inch 300-cm exchange-length guidewire (*yellow arrow*). There are two marker bands (*white arrows*). This balloon is frequently used prior to Wingspan stent (Stryker) placement. **(b)** Fluoroscopy, lateral view, showing delivery of a 4.5-mm × 20-mm Wingspan stent system (Stryker). The Wingspan is a self-expanding nitinol stent with an over-the-wire delivery system (*black arrows*).

11.3 Pearls and Pitfalls

• We rarely use the Wingspan stent system in acute stroke from underlying stenosis because of the need to perform balloon and stent exchanges and the low radial force of the Wingspan (► Fig. 11.3).

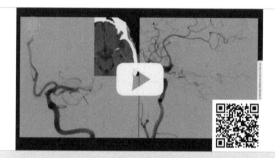

Video 11.1 Failed Angioplasty and Successful Stenting of M2 Occlusion.

• Balloon-mounted stents utilize a rapid-exchange delivery system and offer the option of simultaneous angioplasty and stenting (► Fig. 11.2). However, because of their "stiff" characteristics and limited navigation, robust guide catheter support is needed, sometimes in combination with an intermediate catheter positioned close to the stenosis.

11.4 Cases with Videos and Images

11.4.1 Case 11.1 Failed Angioplasty and Successful Stenting of M2 Occlusion

This case illustrates a clinical scenario of symptomatic middle cerebral artery (MCA) stenosis causing acute stroke that was initially treated with angioplasty alone, followed by emergent stent placement (► **Video 11.1**; ► Fig. 11.4, ► Fig. 11.5, ► Fig. 11.6, ► Fig. 11.7, ► Fig. 11.8, ► Fig. 11.9, ► Fig. 11.10).

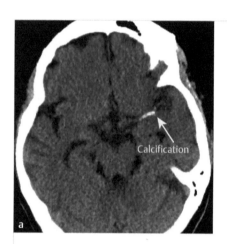

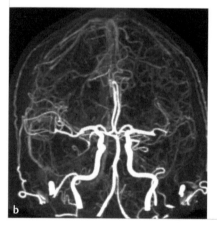

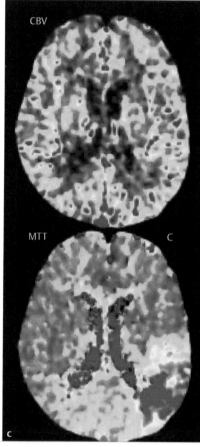

Fig. 11.4 Baseline noninvasive imaging. **(a)** Noncontrast head computed tomography (CT), axial view, with a densely calcified plaque (*arrow*). **(b)** Computed tomographic angiography (CTA), three-dimensional (3D) reconstruction, showing left M2 branch occlusion. **(c)** Computed tomography perfusion (CTP) images showing the corresponding left middle cerebral artery (MCA) territory at risk: preserved cerebral blood volume (CBV; top) and increased mean transit time (MTT; bottom).

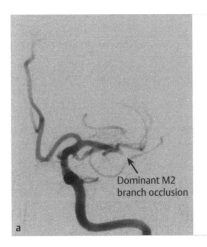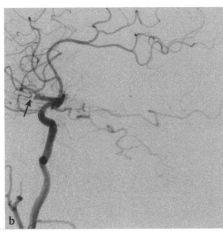

Dominant M2
branch occlusion

a

b

Fig. 11.5 Baseline digital subtraction angiogram (DSA). (a) DSA, anteroposterior (AP) view and (b) lateral view, left internal carotid artery (ICA) injection, showing dominant left M2 branch occlusion (*arrow* in each image).

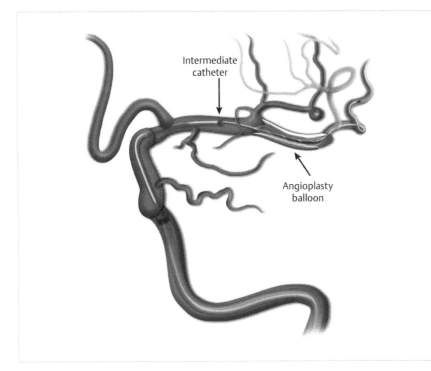

Intermediate
catheter

Angioplasty
balloon

Fig. 11.6 Artist's illustration of balloon angioplasty. The intermediate catheter is navigated into the left M1 middle cerebral artery (MCA) segment, which allows excellent control of the balloon's position. (© Thieme/Jennifer Pryll)

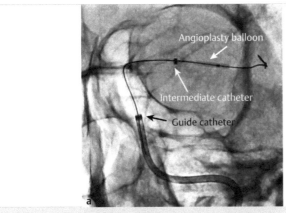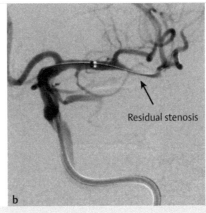

Angioplasty balloon

Intermediate catheter

Guide catheter

a

Residual stenosis

b

Fig. 11.7 Middle cerebral artery (MCA) balloon angioplasty. (a) Fluoroscopy, anteroposterior (AP) view, showing the use of a triaxial system consisting of a guide catheter (*black arrow*), such as a 0.070-inch Neuron or 0.071 Benchmark (Penumbra); an intermediate catheter (*yellow arrow*), such as a 5-French (F) Sofia (MicroVention) or 0.058 Navien (Medtronic); and an angioplasty balloon system (*white arrow*), such as Sprinter (Medtronic) or Mini Trek (Abbott). Note the location of the intermediate catheter in the M1 segment, close to the area of stenosis. Slow gradual angioplasty, approximately 1 atmosphere every 30 to 60 seconds, is performed. We undersize the balloon to approximately 75% of the parent vessel diameter. (b) Digital subtraction angiogram (DSA), AP view, left internal carotid artery (ICA) injection, showing significant residual stenosis postangioplasty (*arrow*). The guidewire remains in place, allowing rapid exchange and stent placement, if needed.

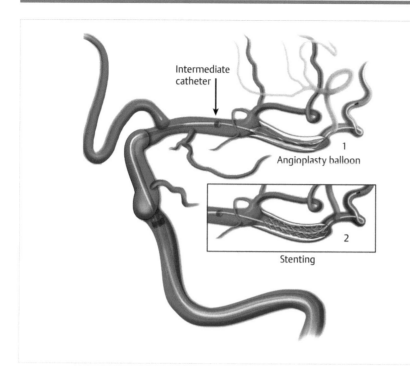

Fig. 11.8 Artist's illustration of rescue stenting. In step 1, angioplasty alone is performed, resulting in significant residual stenosis. In step 2, the angioplasty balloon is removed with the guidewire in place, and a balloon-mounted stent is delivered and deployed. (© Thieme/Jennifer Pryll)

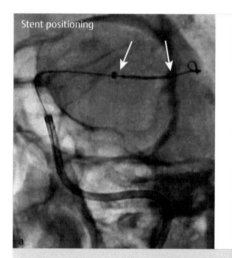

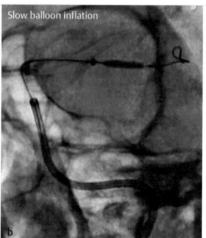

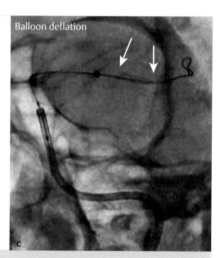

Fig. 11.9 Middle cerebral artery (MCA) stenting. **(a)** Fluoroscopy, high magnification, working projection, showing delivery of a balloon-mounted Resolute Onyx stent (*arrows*; Medtronic). **(b)** Fluoroscopy, also high magnification, showing balloon inflation. **(c)** Fluoroscopy, following balloon deflation. The stent is now fully deployed (*arrows*).

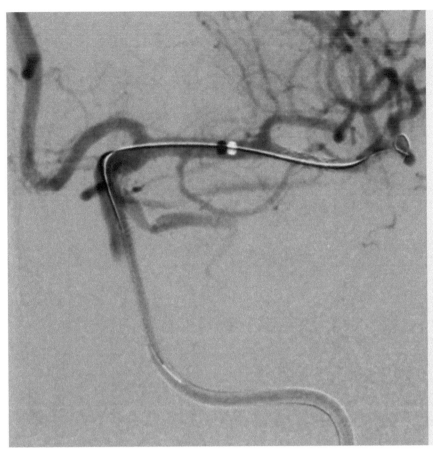

Fig. 11.10 Digital subtraction angiogram (DSA) after middle cerebral artery (MCA) stenting. DSA, anteroposterior (AP) view, showing excellent revascularization of the M2 stenosis. Now it is safe to remove the guidewire and finish the case.

11.4.2 Case 11.2 Fractional Flow Reserve and Primary Stenting of Critical MCA Stenosis

This case illustrates the use of fractional flow reserve (FFR) to estimate the hemodynamic nature of middle cerebral artery (MCA) stenosis and assist in selecting the most appropriate treatment strategy (▶ **Video 11.2**; ▶ Fig. 11.11, ▶ Fig. 11.12, ▶ Fig. 11.13, ▶ Fig. 11.14, ▶ Fig. 11.15).

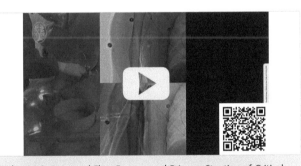

Video 11.2 Fractional Flow Reserve and Primary Stenting of Critical MCA Stenosis.

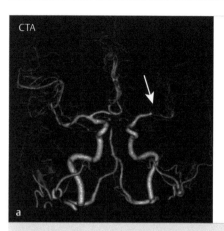
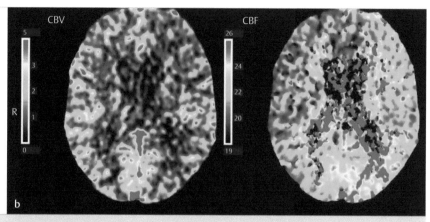

Fig. 11.11 Baseline noninvasive imaging. **(a)** Computed tomographic angiography (CTA), three-dimensional (3D) reconstruction, with left middle cerebral artery (MCA) M1 stenosis (*arrow*). **(b)** Computed tomography perfusion (CTP) images show the corresponding left MCA territory perfusion deficit: cerebral blood volume (CBV; center), mean transit time (MTT; right).

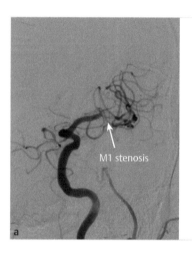
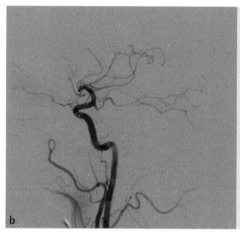

Fig. 11.12 Baseline digital subtraction angiogram (DSA). **(a)** DSA, anteroposterior (AP) and **(b)** lateral views, showing critical left middle cerebral artery (MCA) M1 stenosis (*arrow* in **a**). Note the "isolated MCA" anatomical variant, as the left anterior cerebral artery does not fill on this injection.

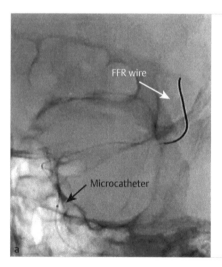
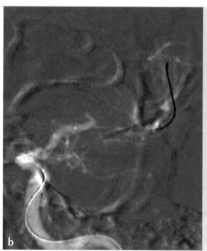

Fig. 11.13 Using a fractional flow reserve (FFR) wire. **(a)** Fluoroscopy and **(b)** roadmap, left internal carotid artery (ICA) injection, antero-posterior (AP) view, showing placement of a 0.014-inch pressure wire (*white arrow*; PrimeWire Prestige Plus [Volcano]) beyond the M1 stenosis. Measuring FFR using pressure wires allows assessment of the functional degree of stenosis and instant evaluation of the adequacy of treatment. Because currently available pressure wires are rather stiff for the delicate intracranial circulation, we prefer first crossing the lesion with a low-profile microcatheter (*black arrow*), such as a Headway Duo (MicroVention) or an SL-10 (Stryker), and a soft guidewire, such as a .014-inch Synchro (Stryker), and then deliver the FFR wire through the microcatheter.

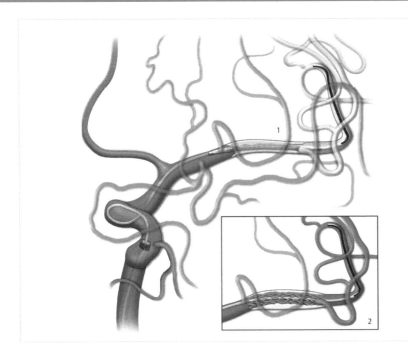

Fig. 11.14 Artist's illustration of stenting using a fractional flow reserve (FFR) wire. In step 1, the FFR wire is used to deliver a balloon-mounted stent. In step 2, once the stent is deployed, a repeat measurement of FFR is performed to ensure that adequate flow is achieved and no further intervention, such as repeat angioplasty or a second stent placement, is needed. (© Thieme/Jennifer Pryll)

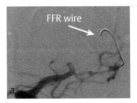

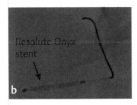

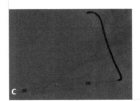

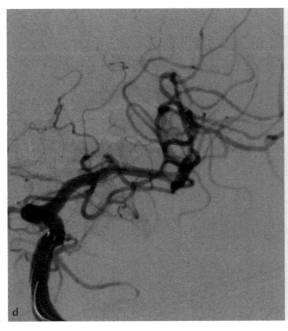

Fig. 11.15 Left middle cerebral artery (MCA) stenting. (a) Digital subtraction angiogram (DSA), anteroposterior (AP) view, showing left MCA stenosis with the fractional flow reserve (FFR) wire (arrow; PrimeWire Prestige Plus [Volcano]) delivered beyond the M1 stenosis. (b) Fluoroscopy, AP view, showing delivery of balloon-mounted Resolute Onyx stent (arrow; Medtronic) at the maximal area of stenosis. (c) Fluoroscopy, AP view, now showing a fully deployed stent. (d) DSA, AP view, left internal carotid artery (ICA) injection, poststent placement. Robust contrast opacification of the left MCA is present.

12 Distal Middle Cerebral Artery Occlusion

General Description

Distal middle cerebral artery (MCA) occlusion, also known as medium vessel occlusion (MeVO), is typically referred to as distal M2 and M3 MCA branch occlusion. Similar to isolated anterior or posterior cerebral artery occlusion strokes, patients with distal MCA occlusions are mainly excluded from endovascular stroke trials and registries. Patients with distal MCA occlusions often present with less severe deficits than "traditional" large vessel occlusion strokes, whereas technically, these cases are often more challenging, given the more distal location of the clot, more fragile vessels, and thus, an increased risk for complications.

Keywords: Middle cerebral artery, aspiration, stent retriever

12.1 Anatomical and Imaging Aspects

- The clinical symptoms associated with an acute distal MCA occlusion could be more difficult to correctly identify as an acute stroke, and radiographic localization of distal MCA occlusion can be challenging. Multimodal noninvasive imaging may alert the interventionist about the presence of distal MCA (▶ Fig. 12.1).
- The benefit of distal MCA thrombectomy should be carefully weighed against the risk of vessel injury (▶ Fig. 12.2). The severity of the patient's symptoms, presence of salvageable brain tissue, and straightforwardness of arterial access should be considered on a case-by-case basis.

12.2 Technique and Key Steps

- Some operators prefer direct aspiration (▶ Fig. 12.3), whereas others rely on stent-retriever (SR) thrombectomy (▶ Fig. 12.4) as the first-line treatment for distal MCA cases. With either approach, smaller profile devices are usually chosen.
- Pharmacological thrombolysis with intra-arterial (IA) alteplase (recombinant tissue plasminogen activator [rtPA]) or glycoprotein IIb/IIIa inhibitors represents a reasonable treatment choice (▶ Fig. 12.3, ▶ Fig. 12.5).

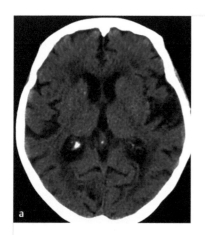
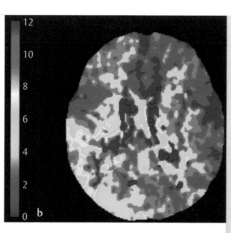
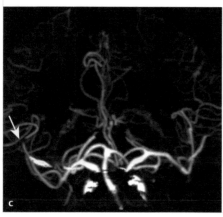
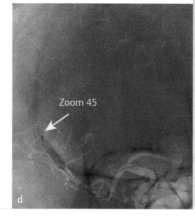

Fig. 12.1 Multimodal imaging of distal middle cerebral artery (MCA) occlusion. **(a)** Noncontrast head computed tomography (CT), axial view. This study is interpreted as "normal" brain CT in a patient with neglect, confusion, and left facial droop but no focal weakness. **(b)** Computed tomography perfusion (CTP) imaging, Tmax sequence, axial view, showing a wedge-shaped perfusion deficit within the right parietal area, raising suspicion for a possible occlusion. **(c)** Computed tomography angiography (CTA) of the head, axial view, confirming a very short drop-off of contrast opacification in one of the right MCA M3 branches (*arrow*), corresponding to the perfusion deficit. Once the diagnosis of acute stroke was made and a MeVO amenable to thrombectomy was confirmed, the patient was taken for emergent thrombectomy. **(d)** Digital subtraction angiography (DSA), roadmap, showing aspiration of the M3 occlusion with a 0.045-inch aspiration catheter (*arrow*; Zoom 45 [Imperative Care]).

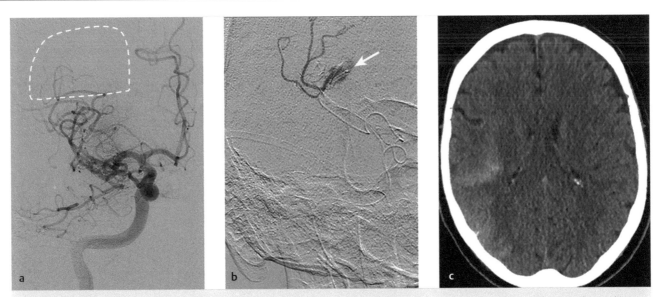

Fig. 12.2 M3 vessel perforation with a microcatheter. **(a)** Digital subtraction angiography (DSA), anteroposterior (AP) view, right internal carotid artery (ICA) injection. Reduced contrast opacification of the superior middle cerebral artery (MCA) trunk territory is present (*highlighted region*), indicating distal MCA occlusion. **(b)** Superselective right MCA injection, showing active contrast extravasation (*arrow*). This could occur while traversing the clot with a guidewire or microcatheter, because distal branches are prone to mechanical injury given their small size. Fortunately, such vessel injury is often self-resolving. **(c)** Noncontrast head computed tomography (CT) postprocedure, showing a minimal amount of contrast material and/or blood products in the right frontoparietal region.

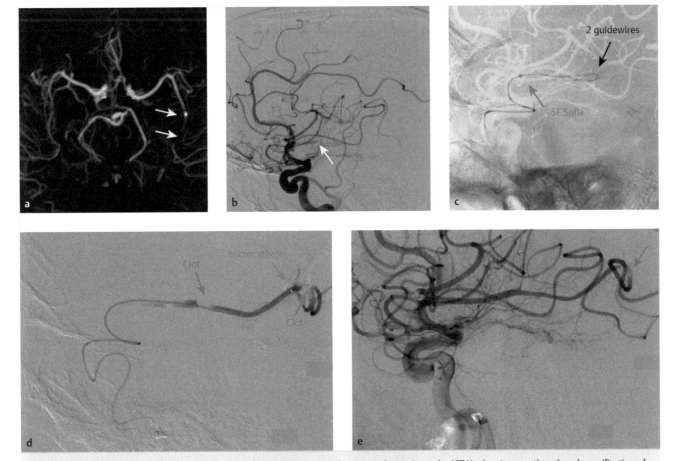

Fig. 12.3 Aspiration thrombectomy of a distal M2 occlusion. **(a)** Computed tomography angiography (CTA), showing greatly reduced opacification of a distal M2 temporal branch on the left side (*arrows*) in comparison to the right side. **(b)** Digital subtraction angiography (DSA), lateral view, confirming distal left M2 inferior trunk occlusion (*arrow*). **(c)** Roadmap, lateral view, showing catheterization of the occluded M2 segment with a 5-French (F) Sofia aspiration catheter (*green arrow*; MicroVention). To help navigate the aspiration catheter, two guidewires (*arrows*; 0.014-inch and 0.010-inch Synchro [Stryker]) are used. **(d)** Superselective left middle cerebral artery (MCA) injection showing distal emboli (*red arrows*). A microcatheter is now placed into the affected M3 branch (*blue arrow*) to slowly inject IIb/IIIa agent Integrilin (eptifibatide). **(e)** DSA, lateral view, repeat injection, confirming near-complete recanalization of the M2 and its more distal territories. A small, nonocclusive residual clot can be seen (*arrow*).

133

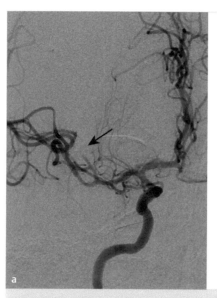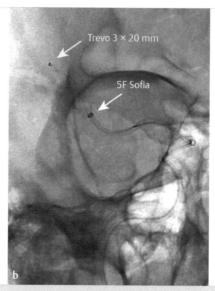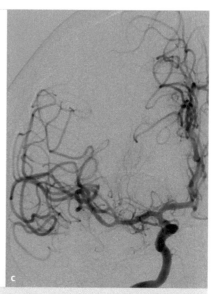

Fig. 12.4 Stent-retriever (SR) thrombectomy of distal M2 occlusion. **(a)** Digital subtraction angiography (DSA), anteroposterior (AP) view, showing distal right middle cerebral artery (MCA) M2 superior trunk occlusion (*arrow*). **(b)** Fluoroscopy, AP view, 3-mm × 20-mm Trevo SR (Stryker) placed distally to the occlusion (*yellow arrow*). In this case, we prefer using a smaller aspiration catheter, such as a 5F Sofia (*white arrow*; MicroVention), to reduce the chance of distal vessel dissection when retrieving the SR. **(c)** DSA, AP view, post-thrombectomy, showing successful recanalization.

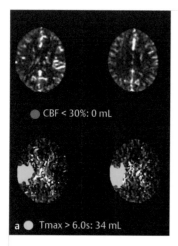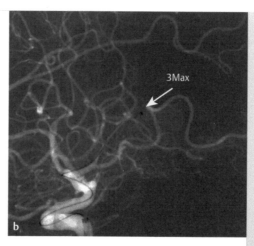

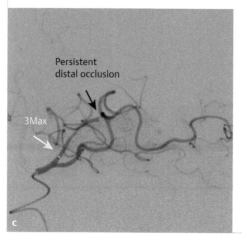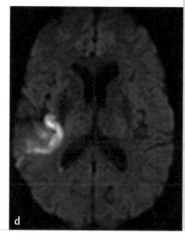

Fig. 12.5 Local thrombolysis of distal middle cerebral artery (MCA) occlusion. **(a)** Computed tomography perfusion (CTP), depicting a distal right MCA territory region with abnormal perfusion (*green*—ischemic penumbra; *magenta*—tissue with greatly reduced CBF, indicative of ischemic core). **(b)** Roadmap, right internal carotid artery (ICA) injection, lateral view, showing access to the occluded M3 segment with a 3Max distal aspiration catheter (*arrow*; Penumbra). **(c)** Digital subtraction angiography (DSA), lateral view, demonstrating persistent occlusion of the affected MCA branch (*black arrow*). Next, 4 mg of recombinant tissue plasminogen activator (rtPA) is slowly infused through the 3Max catheter (*yellow arrow*). **(d)** Magnetic resonance imaging (MRI), diffusion-weighted image, obtained the following day, showing a small residual infarct.

12.3 Cases with Videos and Images

12.3.1 Case 12.1 Stent Retriever for M3 Occlusion

A patient presents with isolated right facial droop, dysarthria, and right arm weakness (▶ **Video 12.1**; ▶ Fig. 12.6, ▶ Fig. 12.7, ▶ Fig. 12.8, ▶ Fig. 12.9, ▶ Fig. 12.10).

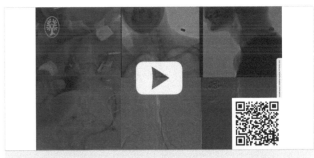

Video 12.1 Stent Retriever for M3 Occlusion.

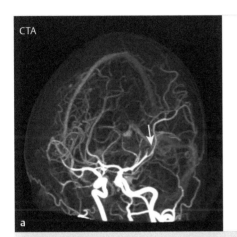
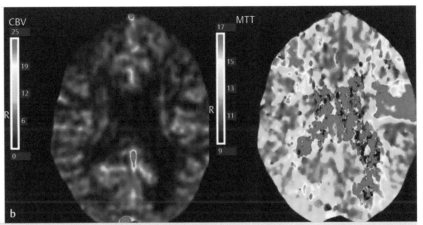

Fig. 12.6 Baseline noninvasive imaging. **(a)** Computed tomography angiography (CTA), three-dimensional (3D) reconstruction, oblique view, showing distal left middle cerebral artery (MCA) (M3 branch) occlusion (*arrow*). **(b)** Computed tomography perfusion (CTP) images show a small perfusion deficit in the left MCA territory, corresponding to the size of the occluded M3 branch. Cerebral blood volume (CBV; left) and prolonged mean transit time (MTT; right).

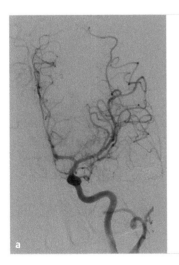
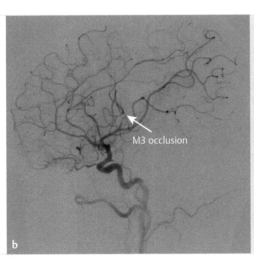

M3 occlusion

Fig. 12.7 Baseline digital subtraction angiography (DSA). **(a)** DSA, left internal carotid artery (ICA) injection, anteroposterior (AP) view. On this projection, all left middle cerebral artery (MCA) branches appear patent. It is difficult to appreciate the occlusion suspected on noninvasive imaging. **(b)** DSA, lateral view, showing left M3 branch occlusion (*arrow*). The lateral view is often needed to detect a distal MCA occlusion.

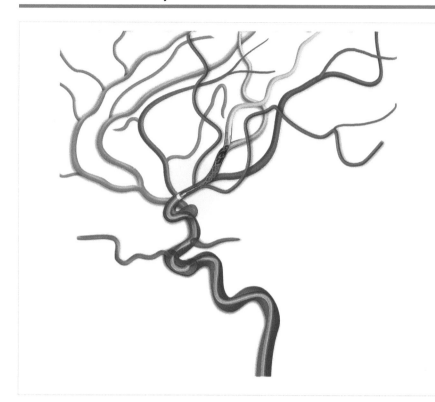

Fig. 12.8 Artist's illustration of distal middle cerebral artery (MCA) stent-retriever (SR) thrombectomy. Artist's drawing demonstrates the value of a small SR and aspiration catheter. A small SR device is chosen that is well suited for a distal occlusion. The aspiration catheter (shown in *green*) allows better control of the micro-catheter when deploying the SR and prevents arterial injury, such as dissection (highlighted region in *yellow*), which could be caused by the SR's pusher wire when the device is being retrieved. (© Thieme/Jennifer Pryll)

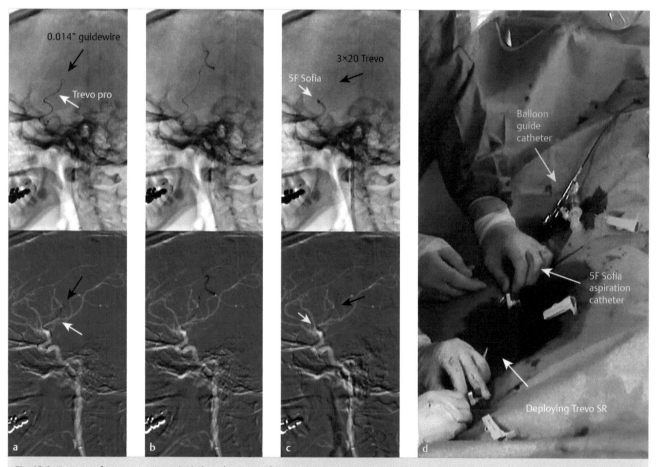

Fig. 12.9 Key steps for stent-retriever (SR) thrombectomy of M3 occlusion. **(a)** Fluoroscopy (*top image*) and roadmap (*bottom image*), lateral views. The occlusion is being traversed with a 0.014-inch guidewire (*black arrow*; Synchro [Stryker]) and 0.021-inch Trevo Pro microcatheter (*white arrow*; Stryker). **(b)** Fluoroscopy (*top image*) and roadmap (*bottom image*), lateral views, showing a microrun performed through the microcatheter to confirm its safe distal position. **(c)** Fluoroscopy (*top image*) and roadmap (*bottom image*), lateral views, showing a 3-mm × 20-mm Trevo SR (*black arrow*; Stryker) and 5F Sofia aspiration catheter (*yellow arrow*; MicroVention). **(d)** Photograph showing deployment of Trevo SR (*white arrow*). The assistant is holding the aspiration catheter (*yellow arrow*). Note that a balloon guide catheter is also used in this case.

12.3.2 Case 12.2 Intra-arterial Thrombolysis for M3/4 Occlusion

This case illustrates the role of local pharmacological thrombolysis when aspiration or stent-retriever (SR) thrombectomy fails or is not feasible (▶ **Video 12.2**; ▶ Fig. 12.11, ▶ Fig. 12.12, ▶ Fig. 12.13, ▶ Fig. 12.14).

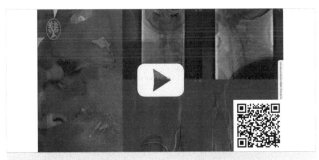

Video 12.2 Intra-arterial Thrombolysis for M3/4 Occlusion.

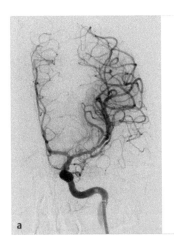
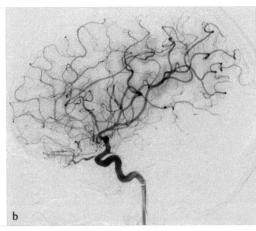

Fig. 12.10 Final digital subtraction angiography (DSA). **(a)** DSA, anteroposterior (AP) view, and **(b)** lateral view, post-MCA (middle cerebral artery) thrombectomy run, showing successful recanalization.

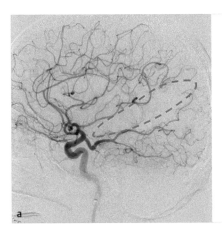
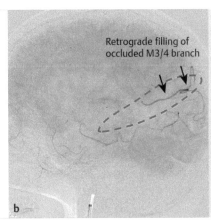

Retrograde filling of occluded M3/4 branch

Fig. 12.11 Baseline digital subtraction angiography (DSA). DSA, left internal carotid artery (ICA) injection, lateral view, **(a)** arterial and **(b)** capillary phases. Very distal occlusions such as the one shown in this case are often difficult to appreciate even with DSA. Careful attention to the capillary phase helps identify a region with decreased contrast opacification (*outlined area*). Retrograde filling of the affected territory via leptomeningeal collaterals is shown (*arrows* in **b**). This is a very distal occlusion, and traditional mechanical thrombectomy approaches are too risky, given the very small size of the affected vessel.

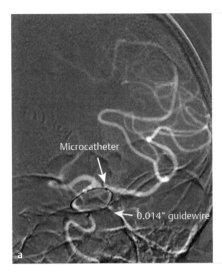
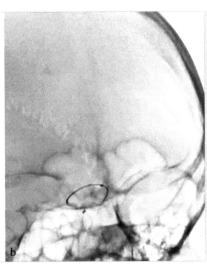

Microcatheter

0.014" guidewire

Fig. 12.12 Accessing target territory with a microcatheter. **(a)** Roadmap and **(b)** fluoroscopy, contralateral oblique view, left internal carotid artery (ICA) injection, showing catheterization of the left middle cerebral artery (MCA) with a microcatheter (Velocity [Penumbra]) and a 0.014-inch guidewire (*arrows* in **a**; Synchro [Stryker]).

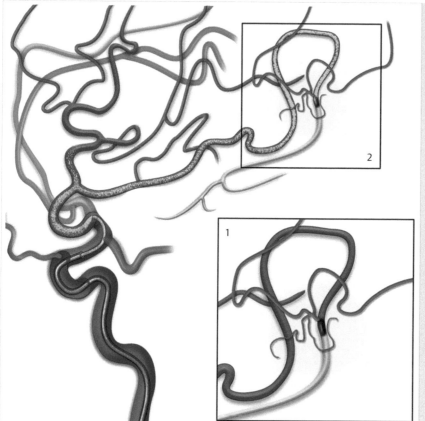

Fig. 12.13 Artist's illustration of pharmacological thrombolysis. Depicted in (1), a very distal left middle cerebral artery (MCA) branch occlusion is present. Such a location would be challenging for mechanical thrombectomy methods that require direct contact with the clot. In (2), the advantage of pharmacological thrombolysis is illustrated; the microcatheter can be positioned more proximally, and the pharmacological agent such as recombinant tissue plasminogen activator (rtPA; depicted in *green*) travels more distally with blood flow, reaching and acting on the clot. (© Thieme/Jennifer Pryll)

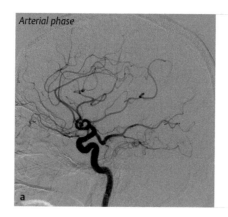

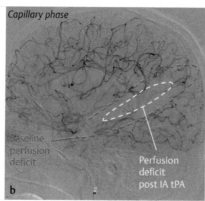

Fig. 12.14 Final digital subtraction angiography (DSA). DSA, left internal carotid artery (ICA) injection, lateral view, **(a)** arterial and **(b)** capillary phases. The *red dashed area* represents the original middle cerebral artery (MCA) perfusion deficit. Note substantially reduced size of perfusion delay after local recombinant tissue plasminogen activator (rtPA) infusion (*yellow dashed area*).

13 Anterior Cerebral Artery Occlusion

General Description

An isolated proximal anterior cerebral artery (ACA) occlusion in a patient presenting with acute ischemic stroke is quite rare. These patients are traditionally excluded from randomized thrombectomy trials, and the frequency of such cases is estimated at approximately 1% according to several interventional registries. More often, ACA occlusion is encountered as a result of embolic complications during carotid angioplasty with or without stenting, as a residual occlusion following intracranial internal carotid artery (ICA) thrombectomy or as a new territory embolization after middle cerebral artery (MCA) thrombectomy. Direct aspiration and stent-retriever (SR) thrombectomy are the main mechanical thrombectomy approaches.

Keywords: anterior cerebral artery, aspiration, emboli of new territories, stent retriever

13.1 Anatomical and Imaging Aspects

- Baseline multimodal noninvasive imaging can be very helpful in diagnosing the presence and extent of ACA occlusion. Intracranial ICA occlusion (ICA-terminus [T] occlusion) will often result in clot extending into the A1 segment while preserving more distal ACA perfusion via the communicating segment. This explains why intracranial ICA occlusions commonly spare the ipsilateral ACA territory on perfusion imaging (▶ Fig. 13.1).
- If residual ACA occlusion is suspected during thrombectomy, a contralateral ICA injection can be performed to distinguish between an "isolated MCA" anatomical variant versus a true ACA occlusion, especially if baseline imaging was insufficient for detailed evaluation of the ACA status at the beginning of the thrombectomy procedure (▶ Fig. 13.2).

13.2 Technique and Key Steps

- Direct aspiration and SR thrombectomy are performed using the same key steps as described in Chapter 9 (Proximal MCA Occlusion—SR Thrombectomy) and Chapter 10 (Proximal MCA Occlusion—Aspiration). For aspiration, because of the

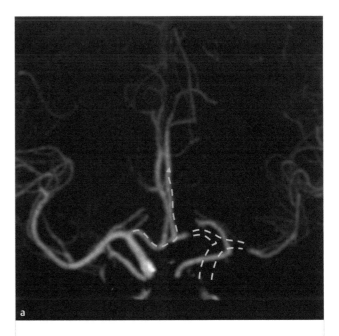

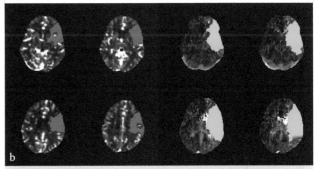

Fig. 13.1 Internal carotid artery-terminus (ICA-T) occlusion with patency of the anterior cerebral artery (ACA) distally. **(a)** Cranial computed tomography angiography (CTA), three-dimensional (3D) reconstruction. The *yellow dashed lines* correspond to the ICA-T filling defect occupied by the clot. Note the preserved opacification of the left ACA beyond the A1 segment as a result of contralateral internal carotid artery (ICA) supply via the anterior communicating artery (*green dashed line*). **(b)** Sequential computed tomography perfusion (CTP) images showing a perfusion deficit within the left middle cerebral artery (MCA) but not the left ACA territory (*purple*—stroke core; *green*—penumbral tissue).

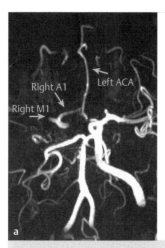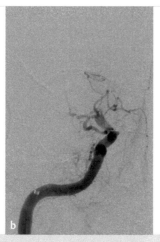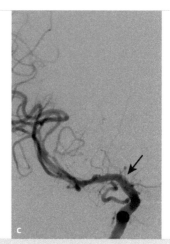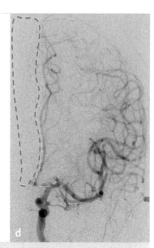

Fig. 13.2 Anterior cerebral artery (ACA) occlusion confirmed during thrombectomy. **(a)** Magnetic resonance angiography (MRA) image showing lack of signal within the right internal carotid artery (ICA) in a case of suspected ICA occlusion. There is opacification of the proximal right M1 and right A1 segment, but no distal right ACA filling. On the basis of the MRA findings alone, it is difficult to precisely understand the extent of the occlusion intracranially. **(b)** Digital subtraction angiography (DSA) image, anteroposterior (AP) view, showing a right internal carotid artery-terminus (ICA-T) occlusion. **(c)** DSA, showing restored patency of the right middle cerebral artery (MCA) after thrombectomy. However, the right ACA does not opacify. There is a subtle filling defect at the origin of the A1 segment that may be due to a clot blocking the A1 takeoff (*arrow*). **(d)** DSA, AP view, contralateral left ICA injection, showing preserved filling of the left ACA territory only (*green dashed territory*). The right ACA does not opacify (*red dashed territory*), suggesting a new right A1 occlusion extending more distally that was not originally present at baseline (based on MRA shown in **a**).

smaller diameter of the ACA in comparison to the MCA, we typically use a smaller aspiration catheter, such as a 0.055-inch 5-French (F) Sofia (MicroVention), 0.054-inch Jet D (Penumbra), or 0.045-inch Zoom 45 (Imperative Care).

- Navigating the aspiration catheter into the ACA segment can be challenging. Using a microcatheter or a second guidewire can help reduce the aspiration catheter catch at the A1 takeoff (► Fig. 13.3).

- For SR thrombectomy, we prefer using a smaller diameter SR device, such as a 3 mm Trevo (Stryker) or an adjustable

diameter SR (Tigertriever [Rapid Medical]). We also use an aspiration catheter for additional proximal aspiration as this reduces the interaction of the SR pusher with the endothelium, minimizing the risk of dissection (► Fig. 13.4).

- For very distal ACA occlusions, we rely on aspiration or pharmacological thrombolysis with intravenous (IV) alteplase (recombinant tissue plasminogen activator [rtPA]) or glycoprotein IIb/IIIa inhibitors (► Fig. 13.4).

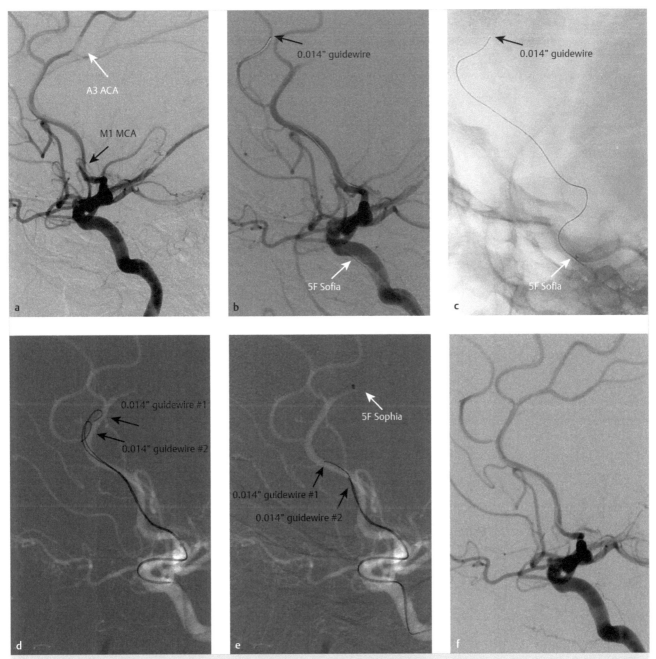

Fig. 13.3 Aspiration thrombectomy of anterior cerebral artery (ACA) occlusion. **(a)** Digital subtraction angiography (DSA), lateral view, showing distal A3 ACA occlusion (*white arrow* points to clot in the pericallosal artery). There is also a separate M1 middle cerebral artery (MCA) occlusion (*black arrow*). **(b)** DSA and **(c)** fluoroscopy, lateral views, showing access to the ACA with a 0.014-inch guidewire (Synchro [Stryker]). The tip of the wire is in the callosomarginal ACA branch (*black arrow*). The *white arrow* points to a 5F Sofia aspiration catheter (MicroVention). The aspiration catheter could not be advanced into the ACA over the guidewire alone. **(d)** Roadmap, lateral view, showing a second 0.014-inch Synchro (Stryker)] guidewire used to catheterize the ACA. This time, both guidewires are navigated into the pericallosal artery (*arrows*). Note the J-shape of the tip; this ensures that the guidewire chooses the largest ACA, often directly following the pathway of the clot. **(e)** Roadmap, lateral view, showing the aspiration catheter successfully reaching the face of the clot (*white arrow*) as the two guidewires are pulled back (*black arrows*). **(f)** DSA, lateral view, demonstrating restored patency of the ACA. This is followed by MCA thrombectomy (not shown).

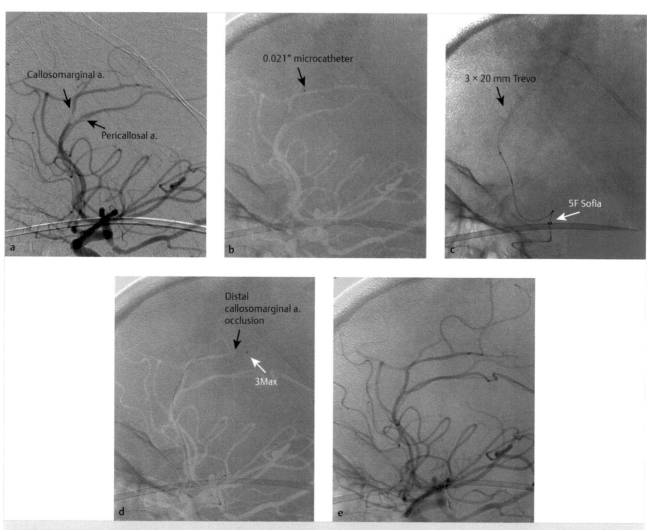

Fig. 13.4 Stent-retriever (SR) thrombectomy of anterior cerebral artery (ACA) occlusion. **(a)** Digital subtraction angiography (DSA), lateral view, showing A2 ACA bifurcation clot extending into the pericallosal and callosomarginal branches (*black arrows*). **(b)** Roadmap, lateral view, showing a 0.021-inch microcatheter (TrevoPro [Stryker]) placed distally to the occlusion into the callosomarginal branch (*arrow*). **(c)** Fluoroscopy showing the SR (*black arrow*; 3 × 20 mm Trevo [Stryker]) and aspiration catheter (*white arrow*; 5F Sofia [MicroVention]). **(d)** Roadmap, lateral view, following SR thrombectomy. A more distal ACA occlusion of the callosomarginal branch is present (*black arrow*). A 0.035-inch distal aspiration catheter (3MAX [Penumbra]) is used for aspiration. **(e)** DSA, lateral view, showing successful aspiration. The ACA is now patent.

13.3 Cases with Videos and Images

13.3.1 Case 13.1 Direct Aspiration of A2 Occlusion

A patient presents with acute onset of severe right hemiparesis. Typically, the affected upper extremity is weaker than the lower extremity. However, in this case, prominent weakness of the right leg was appreciated on examination. The case illustrates isolated middle cerebral artery (MCA) and anterior cerebral artery (ACA) occlusions. The patient received IV alteplase (recombinant tissue plasminogen activator [rtPA]) (▶ **Video 13.1**; ▶ Fig. 13.5, ▶ Fig. 13.6, ▶ Fig. 13.7, ▶ Fig. 13.8, ▶ Fig. 13.9, ▶ Fig. 13.10).

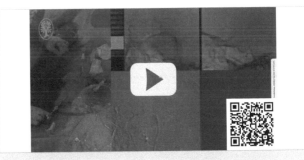

Video 13.1 Direct Aspiration of A2 Occlusion.

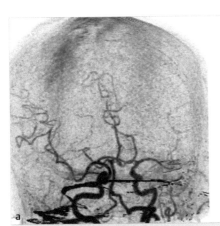
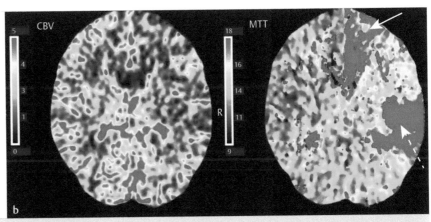

Fig. 13.5 Baseline noninvasive imaging. **(a)** Computed tomography angiography (CTA), three-dimensional (3D) reconstruction, showing somewhat decreased density of the left middle cerebral artery (MCA) branches but no clear proximal occlusion. **(b)** Computed tomography perfusion (CTP) images show the affected territories of the left MCA (*dashed white arrow*) and anterior cerebral artery (ACA) (*solid white arrow*). Cerebral blood volume (CBV; left) and prolonged mean transit time (MTT; right).

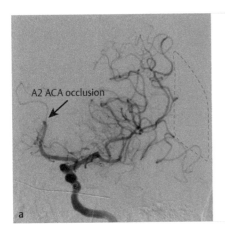
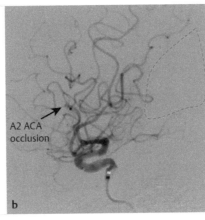

Fig. 13.6 Baseline digital subtraction angiography (DSA). **(a,b)** DSA, left internal carotid artery (ICA) injection, anteroposterior (AP) view, and lateral views, confirming left anterior cerebral artery (ACA) A2 occlusion is present (*arrows*). There is also a subtle distal middle cerebral artery (MCA) occlusion indicated by lack of contrast staining in the outlined territory.

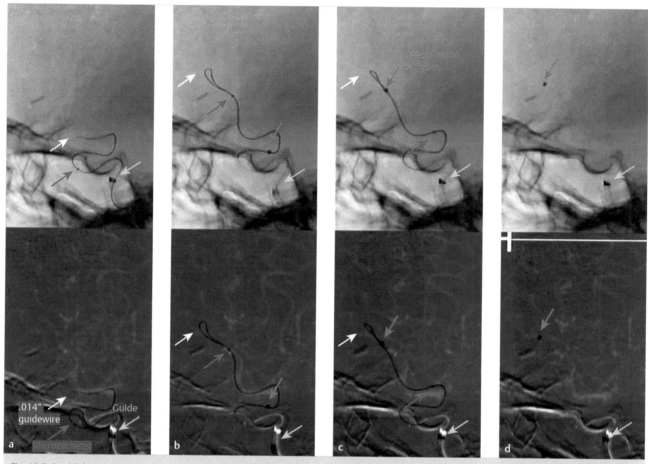

Fig. 13.7 Establishing aspiration catheter access into the anterior cerebral artery (ACA). **(a–d)** Fluoroscopy (*top images*) and roadmap (*bottom images*), lateral views, showing delivery of the Q4 aspiration catheter (MIVI); a microcatheter (0.025-inch Velocity [Penumbra]) and 0.014-inch guidewire are used for delivery. A J-shape is applied to the distal tip of the wire. Q4 system given its (Synchro [Stryker]. Larger internal diameter of Q4 catheter requires microcatheter support whereas the smaller Q3 catheter can be delivered over a guidewire alone. *Yellow arrow*—TrackStar guide catheter [Imperative care], *blue arrow*—Q4 aspiration catheter, *red arrow*—Velocity microcatheter, *white arrow*—Synchro guidewire.

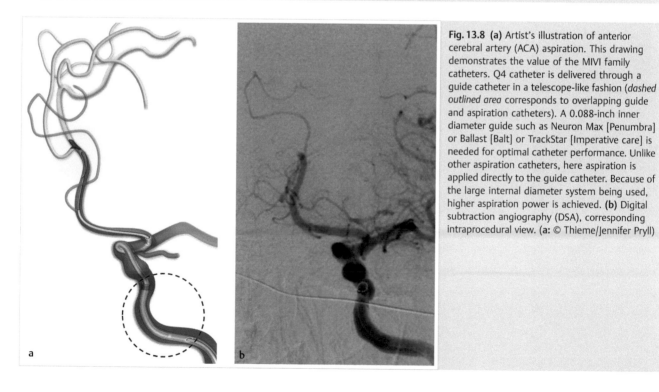

Fig. 13.8 **(a)** Artist's illustration of anterior cerebral artery (ACA) aspiration. This drawing demonstrates the value of the MIVI family catheters. Q4 catheter is delivered through a guide catheter in a telescope-like fashion (*dashed outlined area* corresponds to overlapping guide and aspiration catheters). A 0.088-inch inner diameter guide such as Neuron Max [Penumbra] or Ballast [Balt] or TrackStar [Imperative care] is needed for optimal catheter performance. Unlike other aspiration catheters, here aspiration is applied directly to the guide catheter. Because of the large internal diameter system being used, higher aspiration power is achieved. **(b)** Digital subtraction angiography (DSA), corresponding intraprocedural view. (**a**: © Thieme/Jennifer Pryll)

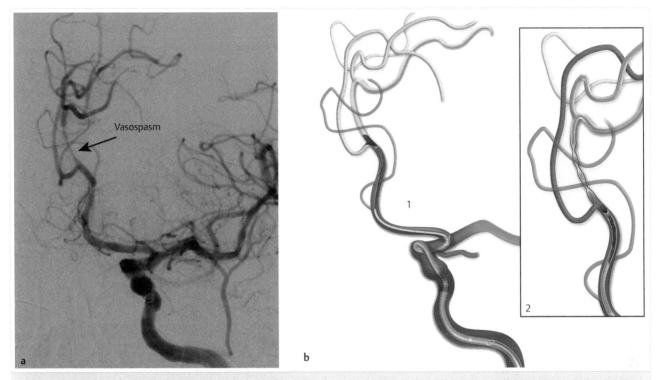

Fig. 13.9 Management of vasospasm after thrombectomy. **(a)** Digital subtraction angiography (DSA), anteroposterior (AP) view, left internal carotid artery (ICA) injection, showing successful recanalization of the left anterior cerebral artery (ACA) after a single aspiration pass. Focal vasospasm (*arrow*) likely as a result of earlier aspiration catheter placement is seen. **(b)** Artist's illustration showing occluded ACA A2 segment and a guidewire, microcatheter, and Q4 aspiration catheter navigated toward the occlusion (1). Following clot aspiration with the Q4 catheter, focal ACA vasospasm is recognized. This can be effectively treated with intravenous (IV) infusion of 5-10 mg of verapamil. (**b**: © Thieme/Jennifer Pryll)

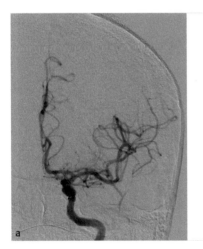
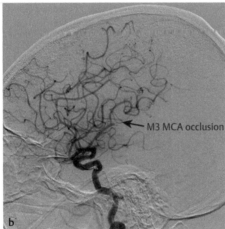

Fig. 13.10 Digital subtraction angiography (DSA) after anterior cerebral artery (ACA) thrombectomy and verapamil administration. DSA, **(a)** anteroposterior (AP), and **(b)** lateral views, showing excellent revascularization of the ACA occlusion. No residual vasospasm is present. A distal M3 middle cerebral artery (MCA) occlusion can be appreciated on the lateral view (*arrow*). This is amenable to aspiration thrombectomy or a small stent-retriever (SR) device (not shown).

13.3.2 Case 13.2 Stent-Retriever Thrombectomy of A2 Occlusion

This patient had sudden onset of profound right hemiparesis and neglect. In this case, an isolated proximal A2 anterior cerebral artery (ACA) occlusion is treated with stent retriever (SR) plus aspiration thrombectomy (▶ **Video 13.2**; ▶ Fig. 13.11, ▶ Fig. 13.12, ▶ Fig. 13.13, ▶ Fig. 13.14).

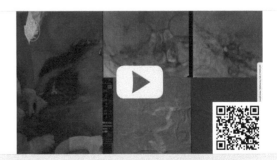

Video 13.2 Stent-Retriever Thrombectomy of A2 Occlusion.

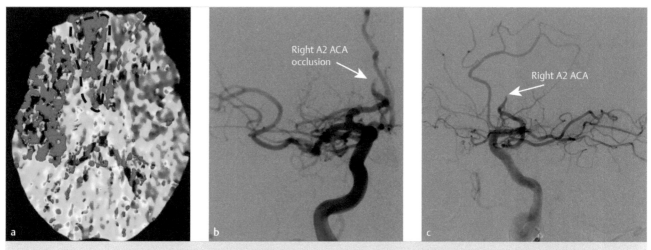

Fig. 13.11 Baseline noninvasive imaging and digital subtraction angiography (DSA). **(a)** Computed tomography perfusion (CTP) image shows a distinct perfusion deficit in the right anterior cerebral artery (ACA) territory (outlined by the *dashed region*) suggesting right ACA occlusion. **(b,c)** DSA, antero-posterior (AP), and lateral views, showing proximal right A2 ACA occlusion (*white arrows*). Opacification of the contralateral left ACA is seen.

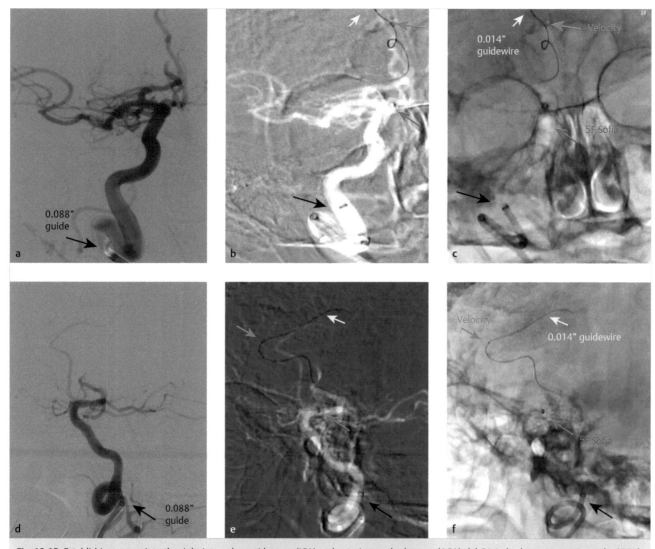

Fig. 13.12 Establishing access into the right internal carotid artery (ICA) and anterior cerebral artery (ACA). **(a)** Digital subtraction angiography (DSA), **(b)** roadmap, and **(c)** fluoroscopy, anteroposterior (AP) view, right ICA injection showing access to the occluded A2 ACA segment. Tortuosity of the right ICA distal cervical segment is appreciated. Triaxial access is chosen, consisting of the 0.088-inch guide catheter (*black arrow*; Neuron Max [Penumbra]), intermediate catheter (*red arrow*; 5F Sofia [MicroVention]), and 0.025-inch microcatheter (*blue arrow*; Velocity [Penumbra]). A 0.014-inch guidewire (*arrow*; Synchro [Stryker]) and the microcatheter have traversed the occlusion site ready for stent-retriever (SR) delivery. **(d)** DSA, **(e)** roadmap, and **(f)** fluoroscopy, lateral view. The *arrow labels* are similar to panels **a–c**.

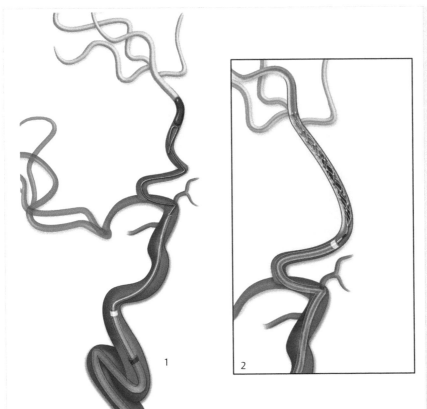

Fig. 13.13 Artist's illustration of anterior cerebral artery (ACA) stent-retriever (SR) thrombectomy. The initial attempt is made to advance the aspiration catheter into the ACA over guidewire/microcatheter alone without crossing the clot (highlighted region in *yellow*). However, attempts to deliver the aspiration catheter any further are unsuccessful (1). This time, SR is planned. The lesion is crossed with guidewire/microcatheter and once the SR is unsheathed, the aspiration catheter is brought all the way to the proximal end of the clot (2). (© Thieme/Jennifer Pryll)

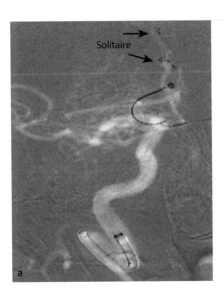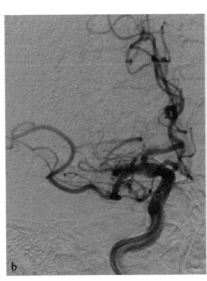

Fig. 13.14 Anterior cerebral artery (ACA) stent-retriever (SR) thrombectomy. **(a)** Roadmap, anteroposterior (AP) view, showing 4 × 20 mm Solitaire (Medtronic) unsheathed within the right ACA (*black arrows*). The aspiration catheter is now brought into the right ACA A2 segment, pinning the proximal end of the clot (*red arrow*). **(b)** Digital subtraction angiography (DSA), AP view, post ACA thrombectomy run, showing successful recanalization of the right ACA. Right M2 middle cerebral artery (MCA) SR thrombectomy is performed next (not shown).

14 Vertebral Artery Occlusion

General Description

Vertebral artery (VA) occlusion as a cause of acute stroke can present as an isolated lesion located either at the VA origin (often as a result of underlying atherosclerotic disease) or more distally (mainly as a result of VA dissection). VA stenosis or occlusion can also be encountered in strokes caused by a tandem lesion, where a more distal basilar artery (BA) occlusion is present.

Keywords: balloon-mounted stent, dissection, drug-eluting stent, ostial lesion

14.1 Anatomical and Imaging Aspects

- There are four distinct segments that are commonly used for anatomical classification of the VA: V1 (preforaminal segment), V2 (foraminal segment), V3 (atlantic segment), and V4 (intracranial segment) (► Fig. 14.1).
- Atherosclerosis is the most common cause of VA origin occlusion or flow-limiting stenosis. Computed tomography

angiography (CTA) or magnetic resonance angiography (MRA) may underestimate or overestimate the degree of VA stenosis. With a high index of clinical suspicions for VA causing flow-related phenomenon, even with patency of the BA seen on noninvasive imaging, emergent catheter angiography should be considered (► Fig. 14.2).

- On cervical CTA, VA origin lesion can be difficult to visualize due to artifact from contrast material in the subclavian vein, which can occur as a result of incorrect timing of the venous contrast injection or due to poor cardiac output (► Fig. 14.3).
- The VA should not be mistaken for a prominent appearance of the deep cervical artery (► Fig. 14.4).
- Dissection should be suspected in cases of a more distally located VA occlusion (► Fig. 14.5).
- For cases of internal carotid artery (ICA) occlusion in which the posterior circulation also provides significant supply to the affected territory, VA stenting can be used to augment intracranial flow. Computed tomography perfusion (CTP) imaging often helps the neurointerventionist establish the territory at risk and evaluate changes in flow following intervention (► Fig. 14.6).

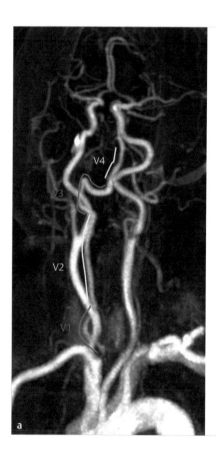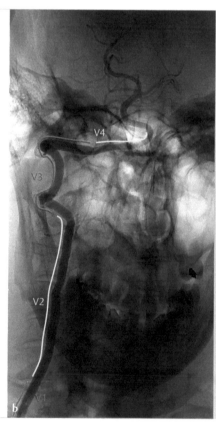

Fig. 14.1 Vertebral artery (VA) segments. **(a)** Craniocervical magnetic resonance angiography (MRA), anteroposterior (AP) view, in a patient with severe stenosis of the right VA origin. The left VA artery is severely hypoplastic. V1 (preforaminal segment) begins at the VA origin and commonly enters the transverse foramen of C6. V2 (foraminal segment) follows the transverse foramen to C2. V3 (atlantic segment) is from C2 to the dura. V4 (intracranial segment) joins the contralateral VA to form the basilar artery (BA). **(b)** Right VA injection, AP view. V1–V4 segments are shown.

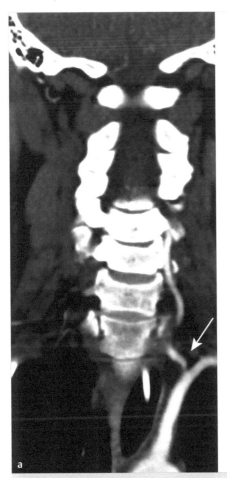
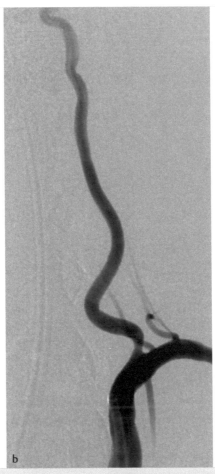
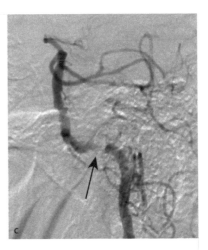
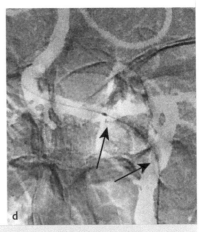

Fig. 14.2 Vertebral artery (VA) stenosis misdiagnosed on computed tomography angiography (CTA). **(a)** CTA, coronal view, with suspected flow-limiting origin stenosis (*arrow*) in a patient with posterior circulation acute stroke. **(b)** Digital subtraction angiogram (DSA), anteroposterior (AP) view, showing only 50% stenosis of the left VA origin. This alone would not result in flow limiting stenosis. **(c)** DSA, oblique projection, intracranial view, showing a critical short-segment flow-limiting stenosis of the left vertebrobasilar junction (*arrow*), causing the stroke symptoms. **(d)** Roadmap showing angioplasty of this flow-limiting stenosis. The *arrows* point to the proximal and distal markers of a noncompliant coronary balloon.

14.2 Techniques and Key Steps

- Severe subclavian artery (SA) tortuosity is frequently encountered. Radial artery access, approaching from the right or left side, depending on which VA is affected, is often preferable.
- If femoral artery access is used, we prefer a "stiffer" type guide catheter such as a 0.070-inch Envoy (Codman) or a long sheath (6-French [F] Cook shuttle [Cook Medical]). A "buddy" wire such as a 0.018-inch V18 guidewire (Boston Scientific) can be used for extra support (▶ Fig. 14.6).
- For VA origin stenosis, balloon-mounted coronary stents are our first choice (▶ Fig. 14.6). They provide the advantages of a

rapid-exchange system, thus only requiring a 200-cm guidewire (we prefer 0.014-inch guidewires with extra support such as Transcend [Stryker] or Spartacore [Abbott]) and sufficient radial force required to treat highly calcified plaques. In addition, such stents allow simultaneous angioplasty and stent deployment, thus minimizing the risk of embolization, since distal embolic protection devices, such as filters, are usually not used in the VA.
- Bare-metal stents require 3 months of dual antiplatelet therapy (DAPT), whereas drug-eluting stents (DES) typically require 12 months of DAPT.
- Underlying dissection is best treated with intracranial stents such as the Neuroform Atlas (Stryker) or Enterprise (Codman) (▶ Fig. 14.5).

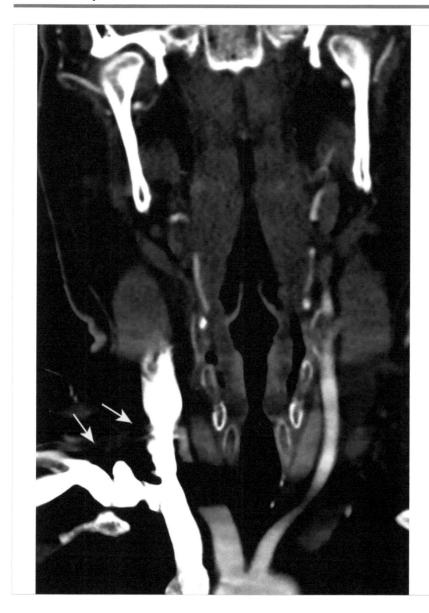

Fig. 14.3 Streak artifact on computed tomography angiography (CTA). Cervical CTA, coronal view, showing significant streak artifact from iodine contrast material in the right subclavian artery (SA) and jugular veins (*arrows*). Thus, evaluation of the right vertebral artery (VA) origin in this case is limited.

14.3 Pearls and Pitfalls

- If predilatation is needed, compliant intracranial balloons (such as HyperGlide [Medtronic] or TransForm [Stryker]) should be avoided; they will not generate enough force for sufficient angioplasty, yet can rupture the VA distally to the stenosis. Instead, noncompliant coronary angioplasty balloons or a semicompliant Gateway balloon (Stryker) should be used.
- It is a common mistake to aim for a "perfect" landing of the stent when treating VA stenosis by trying to minimize the amount of device overhang or prolapse into the SA, resulting in proximal stent migration and requiring additional stent placement (▶ Fig. 14.7).

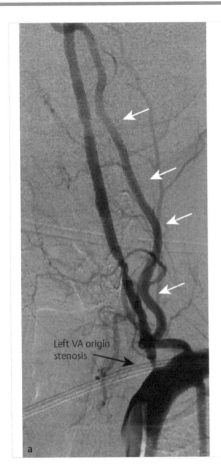
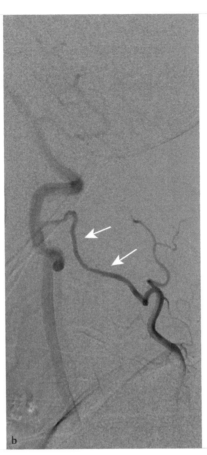

Left VA origin stenosis

Fig. 14.4 Deep cervical artery. (a) Digital subtraction angiogram (DSA), anteroposterior (AP) view, left subclavian artery (SA) injection, showing critical left vertebral artery (VA) origin stenosis (*black arrow*). The stenotic lesion was missed on computed tomography angiography (CTA) because the left VA was mistaken for a prominent appearance of the deep cervical artery (*white arrows*). The deep cervical artery runs parallel to the VA and commonly arises from the costocervical trunk, which is distal to the VA origin. (b) DSA, lateral cranial view, showing the deep cervical artery anastomosing with the VA at its V3 segment (*arrows*).

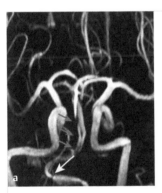
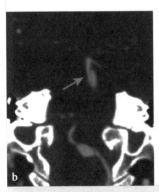
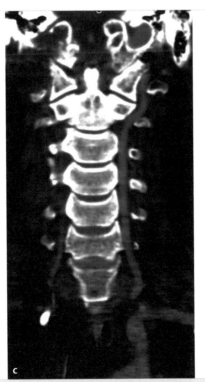
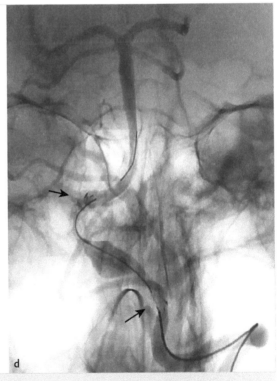

Fig. 14.5 Flow-limiting V4 dissection. (a) Magnetic resonance angiography (MRA), coronal view, showing left vertebral artery (VA) V4 dissection extending into the basilar artery (BA; *red arrows*). Flow-limiting stenosis of the V4 segment is seen (*yellow arrow*), along with a more proximal fusiform pseudoaneurysm. (b) Computed tomography angiography (CTA), coronal cranial view, without any evidence of calcifications, again indicating that dissection, rather than another etiology (such as atherosclerosis), is the underlying etiology in this case. Note that the dissection extends nearly to the very end of the BA (*arrow*). (c) CTA, coronal cervical view, showing patent left VA more proximally. (d) Digital subtraction angiogram (DSA), anteroposterior (AP) view, showing deployment of an intracranial stent (Enterprise [Codman]). The *arrows* point to the proximal and distal stent markers.

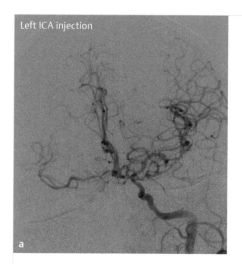
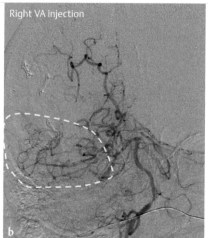
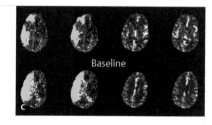
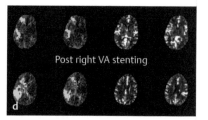
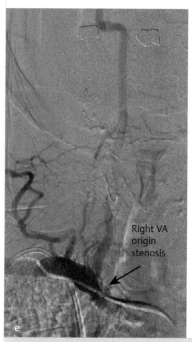
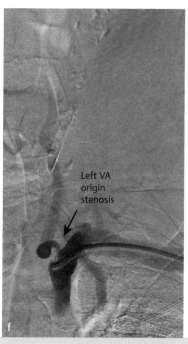
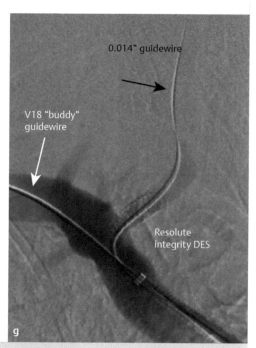

Fig. 14.6 Vertebral artery (VA) origin stenting to augment supply to the anterior circulation. **(a)** Digital subtraction angiogram (DSA), anteroposterior (AP) view, left internal carotid artery (ICA) injection, in a patient with a chronic right ICA occlusion showing only partial opacification of the right middle cerebral artery (MCA) territory. **(b)** DSA, AP view, right VA injection, demonstrating partial contribution to the right MCA territory via right posterior cerebral artery–MCA leptomeningeal collaterals (*outlined area*). **(c)** Computed tomography perfusion (CTP) with a prominent perfusion deficit in the right MCA territory (*green*). **(d)** Following right VA stenting, the right MCA territory perfusion deficit is much smaller (*green*). **(e)** DSA, right subclavian artery (SA) injection, showing severe right VA origin stenosis (*arrow*). **(f)** DSA, left SA injection, with severe left VA origin stenosis (*arrow*). The left VA takeoff appears more tortuous in comparison to the right side; thus, right VA stenting is chosen. **(g)** DSA, right SA injection, demonstrating restored patency of the right VA origin following placement of a balloon-mounted coronary stent (4-mm × 18-mm Resolute Integrity drug-eluting stent [DES; Medtronic]). Note how approximately one-fourth to one-third of the device length extends into the SA. This is done on purpose to prevent proximal device migration (often referred to as "watermelon-seeding" effect). The 0.014-inch guidewire remains in place until DSA confirms optimal state position. An additional guidewire (*white arrow*, V18 "buddy" wire) is used to allow extra support for the guide catheter (6F Cook shuttle [Cook Medical]).

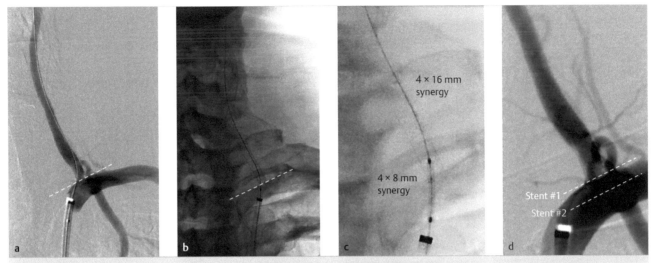

Fig. 14.7 Vertebral artery (VA) origin stent migration. **(a)** Digital subtraction angiogram (DSA) and **(b)** fluoroscopy, anteroposterior (AP) view, showing deployment of a balloon-mounted coronary stent to treat left VA origin stenosis (4 × 16 mm Synergy [Boston Scientific]). The *dashed lines* correspond to the proximal end of the stent, which is best appreciated on the fluoroscopy image. **(b)** Shortly after stent deployment, proximal migration of the stent was noted. **(c)** Fluoroscopy, AP view, showing delivery of a second stent (another 4-mm × 8-mm Synergy) to create an overlap with the first device. This illustrates the importance of keeping the guidewire in place until angiography confirms a satisfactory procedural result. Reaccessing a freshly placed stent can further cause device migration and/or deformation. **(d)** DSA, left subclavian artery (SA), following second stent deployment. The *white* and *yellow dashed lines* correspond to the proximal ends of the first and second stents, respectively. Extending the stent into the SA prevents proximal stent migration.

14.4 Cases with Videos and Images

14.4.1 Case 14.1 Vertebral Artery Origin Stenting and Ostial Balloon Angioplasty

In this case, flow-limiting left vertebral artery (VA) origin stenosis was diagnosed on emergent noninvasive imaging in a patient with acute onset of ataxia, diplopia, and dysarthria. The right VA was not visualized (▶ **Video 14.1**; ▶ Fig. 14.8, ▶ Fig. 14.9, ▶ Fig. 14.10, ▶ Fig. 14.11, ▶ Fig. 14.12).

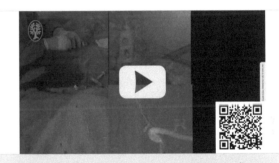

Video 14.1 Vertebral Artery Origin Stenting and Ostial Balloon Angioplasty.

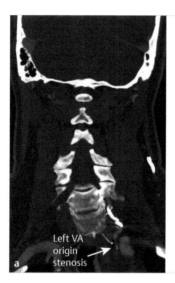
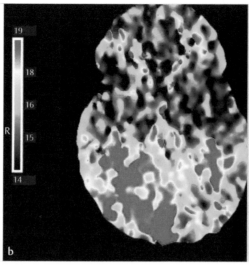

Fig. 14.8 Baseline imaging obtained on the patient's presentation to the emergency department. **(a)** Cervical computed tomography angiography (CTA), coronal view, demonstrating severe left vertebral artery (VA) origin stenosis (*arrow*). Focal hyperdensity indicative of calcifications can be appreciated. **(b)** Computed tomography perfusion (CTP) image showing increased time-to-peak (TTP) in the posterior fossa territory.

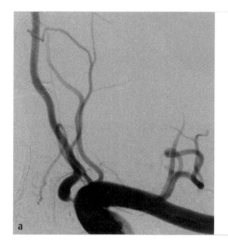
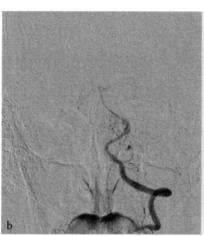

Fig. 14.9 Baseline digital subtraction angiogram (DSA). **(a)** Left subclavian artery (SA) injection, anteroposterior (AP) view, confirming critical left vertebral artery (VA) origin stenosis. **(b)** Left SA injection, intracranial view, with diminished filling of the basilar artery (BA) and its branches, indicating the flow-limiting nature of the stenosis.

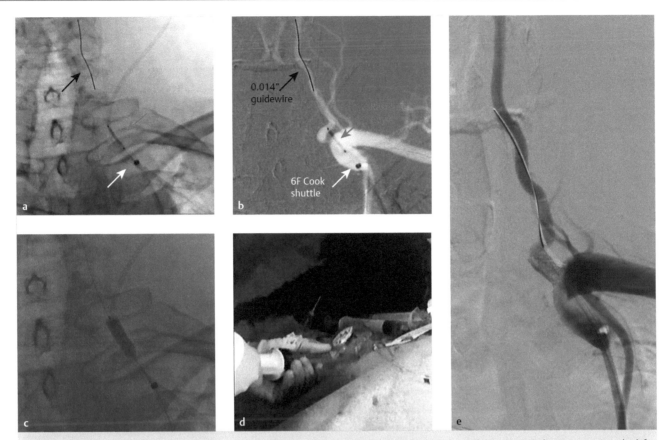

Fig. 14.10 Access through the lesion and stent placement. **(a)** Fluoroscopy (*top image*) and **(b)** roadmap (*bottom image*) showing access to the left vertebral artery (VA) with a 0.014-inch guidewire (*black arrow*; Spartacore [Abbott]) and delivery of a Resolute Onyx (*red arrow*) balloon-mounted stent (Medtronic) through the lesion. The stent has proximal and distal radiopaque markers to facilitate accurate stent delivery. A 6F Cook shuttle (Cook Medical) guide catheter is used (*white arrow*). **(c)** Fluoroscopy showing balloon inflation. **(d)** Photograph showing operator's use of the inflation device. These devices allow controlled balloon inflation and deflation to ensure that pressure does not rise above the balloon's burst pressure. **(e)** Digital subtraction angiogram (DSA), left subclavian artery (SA) injection, confirming successful stent placement.

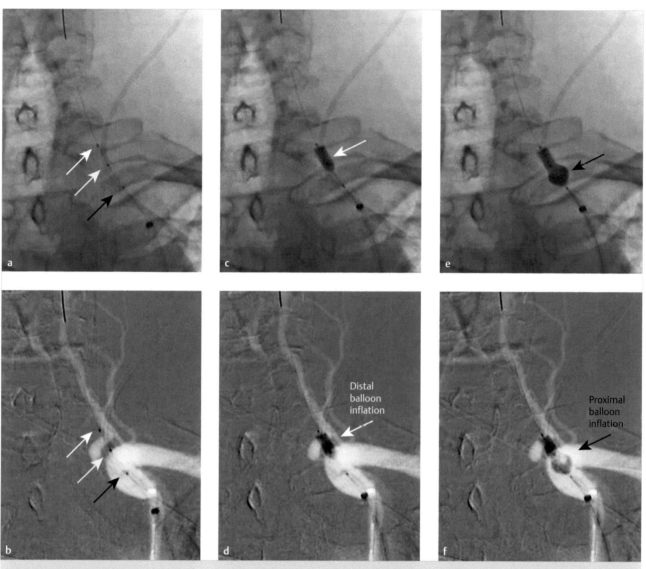

Fig. 14.11 Use of the Ostial FLASH dual balloon system (Ostial Corporation/Cardinal Health). **(a)** Fluoroscopy (*top image*) and **(b)** roadmap (*bottom image*) showing delivery of the ostial FLASH dual balloon. The rapid exchange system allows easy removal of the balloon-mounted stent and delivery of the FLASH balloon over the guidewire. The three marker bands are the distal marker (*white arrows*); the middle marker (*yellow arrows*), which is at the ostium; and the proximal marker (*black arrows*), which should be positioned outside of the guide catheter. **(c)** Fluoroscopy (*top image*) and **(d)** roadmap (*bottom image*) showing inflation of the proximal noncompliant balloon (*arrow*). This is done using an inflation (indeflator) device. **(e)** Fluoroscopy (*top image*) and **(f)** roadmap (*bottom image*) showing inflation of the compliant, low-pressure proximal balloon (*arrow*). Inflation is accomplished using a 1-mL syringe. This causes flaring of the proximal edges of the stent.

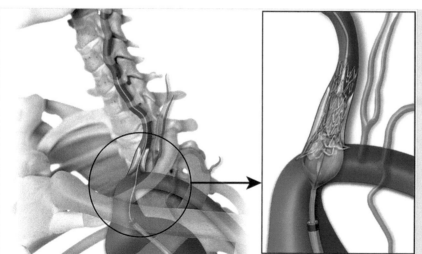

Fig. 14.12 Artist's illustration of the use of an ostial balloon system. The image on the left illustrates critical left vertebral artery (VA) origin stenosis. A guide catheter is placed into the left VA and access with a guidewire through the lesion has been established. The image on the right depicts how the ostial balloon achieves flaring of the stent tines at the proximal end of the stent and optimal wall apposition using its dual balloon design. (© Thieme/Jennifer Pryll)

15 Basilar Artery Occlusion—Mechanical Thrombectomy

General Description

Acute basilar artery (BA) occlusion can present as a wide range of stroke symptoms from mild visual disturbance, gait difficulty, or extremity weakness to coma. The onset can be more insidious, lasting hours to even days; and as a result, posterior circulation strokes can sometimes be mistaken for other diseases. Although the evidence in support of BA thrombectomy is not as robust as that for anterior circulation strokes, the BA and posterior cerebral arteries (PCA) can be effectively treated with the modern thrombectomy approaches to large vessel occlusion (LVO) and medium vessel occlusion (MeVO).

Keywords: basilar artery, posterior cerebral artery, stent retriever

15.1 Anatomical and Imaging Aspects

- Computed tomographic angiography (CTA) or magnetic resonance angiography (MRA) should be performed if acute BA occlusion is suspected. The hyperdense BA sign may or may not be present on noncontrast CT, depending on clot composition, similar to the case with anterior circulation LVO strokes (▶ Fig. 15.1).
- The clinical value of the posterior circulation Alberta Stroke Program Early CT Score (pc ASPECTS) is limited by frequent artifact seen in the posterior fossa. Perfusion imaging is frequently nondiagnostic (▶ Fig. 15.2).

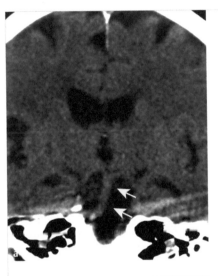
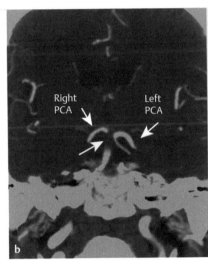
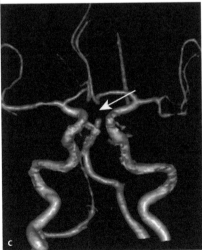
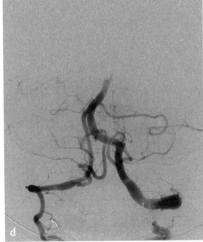

Fig. 15.1 Acute basilar artery (BA) occlusion. (a) Noncontrast head computed tomography (CT), coronal view. Homogeneous appearance of the BA is seen without any distinct hyperdense signal (*arrows*). (b) Computed tomographic angiography (CTA), coronal view, showing a filling defect of the distal BA (*yellow arrow*), consistent with acute BA occlusion. Opacification of both posterior cerebral arteries (PCAs; *white arrows*) is seen as a result of collateral flow through the posterior communicating (PCom) segments. (c) CTA, three-dimensional (3D) reconstruction, also demonstrating top of the BA occlusion (*arrow*). (d) Digital subtraction angiography (DSA), left vertebral artery (VA) injection, confirming BA occlusion.

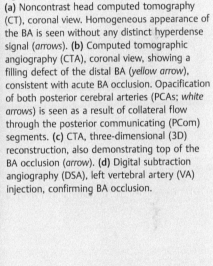

- The appearance of the BA can be extremely variable. Prominent PCA supply from the internal carotid artery (ICA) via its posterior communicating (PCom) segment (so-called "fetal PCA") may be mistaken for an acute top of the BA occlusion (▶ Fig. 15.3).

- An isolated distal PCA occlusion can be difficult to recognize on CTA or MRA alone. Corresponding clinical symptoms, such as contralateral hemianopsia, or a perfusion scan with a deficit corresponding to the PCA territory should trigger careful examination of the PCA in question.

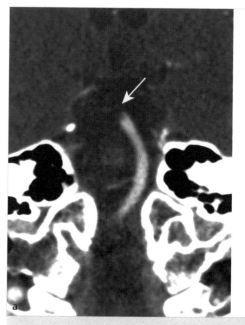
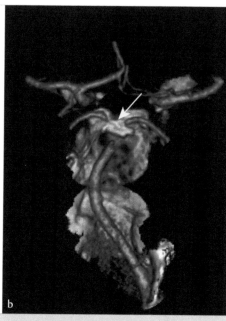
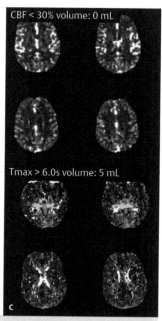

Fig. 15.2 Example of nondiagnostic perfusion imaging in a case of basilar artery (BA) occlusion. Computed tomographic angiography (CTA), **(a)** coronal view and **(b)** three-dimensional (3D) reconstruction, demonstrating top of the BA occlusion (*arrow* in each image). **(c)** Computed tomography perfusion (CTP) imaging, RapidAI (iSchemaView) map, showing nonspecific patchy areas of increased Tmax > 6 seconds (bottom half).

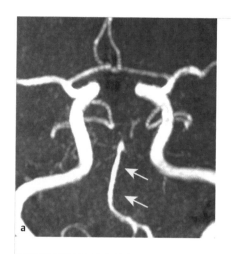
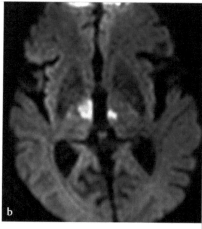

Fig. 15.3 Bilateral fetal posterior cerebral artery (PCA) variant. **(a)** Magnetic resonance angiography (MRA), three-dimensional (3D) reconstruction, showing a hypoplastic basilar artery (BA; *arrows*). Both PCAs are supplied via the internal carotid arteries (ICAs). **(b)** Magnetic resonance imaging (MRI), diffusion-weighted imaging (DWI) sequence, axial view, showing bilateral thalamic infarcts as a result of occlusion of thalamoperforator branches. **(c)** Digital subtraction angiography (DSA), left vertebral artery (VA) injection, anteroposterior (AP) view. Note lack of bilateral PCA opacification. Superior cerebellar arteries (*black arrow*, right superior cerebellar artery [SCA]; *red arrow*, left SCA) and thalamoperforators (*yellow arrows*) are shown. **(d)** DSA, left VA, lateral projection, showing robust opacification of the ipsilateral PCA (*arrows*). Thrombectomy is not indicated in this case.

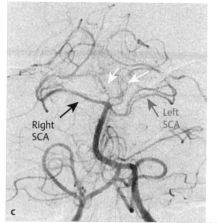
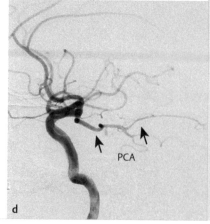

15.2 Techniques and Key Steps

- Radial artery access is often preferable for posterior circulation thrombectomy. Depending on the laterality of the dominant vertebral artery (VA), left radial artery access may be required. Using a long 0.088-inch sheath, such as Ballast (Balt) or Infinity (Stryker), will accommodate most modern aspiration catheters and allow a wide range of thrombectomy choices.

- Direct aspiration (▶ Fig. 15.4) or stent-retriever (SR) thrombectomy (▶ Fig. 15.5) can be used for BA or proximal PCA occlusions.

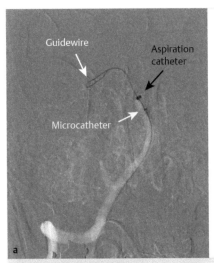
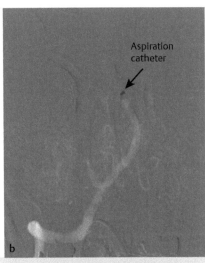
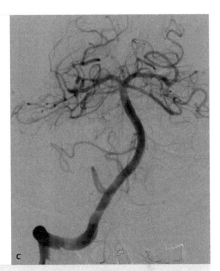

Fig. 15.4 Aspiration thrombectomy of basilar artery (BA) occlusion. (a) Roadmap, right vertebral artery (VA) injection. The occlusion is traversed with a 0.014 guidewire (*white arrow*; Synchro [Stryker]). The 6-French (F) aspiration catheter (*black arrow*; Q6 [MIVI]) is delivered to the clot over a microcatheter (*yellow arrow*; Velocity [Penumbra]). Although traversing the lesion with a guidewire is not ideal because it may result in distal embolization, sometimes this is needed to gain more support while advancing the aspiration catheter. (b) Roadmap, right VA injection. The guidewire and microcatheter have been removed. The aspiration catheter is embedded in the proximal end of the clot (*arrow*). Aspiration is now applied. (c) Digital subtraction angiography (DSA), right VA, post-thrombectomy. Successful recanalization is achieved with aspiration alone.

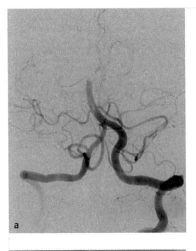
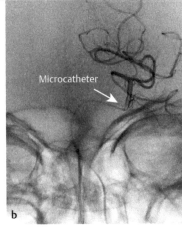

Fig. 15.5 Stent-retriever (SR) thrombectomy of basilar artery (BA) occlusion. (a) Digital subtraction angiography (DSA), anteroposterior (AP) view, left vertebral artery (VA) injection, demonstrating distal BA occlusion. (b) Superselective microcatheter injection of the left posterior cerebral artery (PCA) after traversing the occlusion. The *arrow* points to the tip of the microcatheter (Velocity [Penumbra]). Safe position of the microcatheter prior to SR delivery and unsheathing is confirmed. (c) Fluoroscopy showing deployed SR (4 × 20 mm Trevo [Stryker]). *Arrow* points to a 0.068-inch intermediate catheter used for aspiration (ACE 68 [Penumbra]). (d) DSA, left VA, post-thrombectomy, showing successful recanalization.

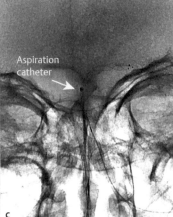
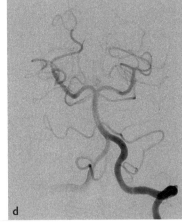

15.3 Pearls and Pitfalls

- Given anatomical variations in the size and presence or absence of the PCA P1 and ICA PCom segments, an atretic or hypoplastic P1 segment should not be confused with an acutely occluded P1 segment (▶ Fig. 15.6).

- For more distal PCA occlusions, we prefer aspiration with a smaller caliber catheter, such as a 0.035-inch 3MAX (Penumbra) or Zoom 35 (Imperative Care) (▶ Fig. 15.7), or local pharmacological thrombolysis.

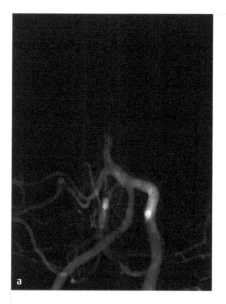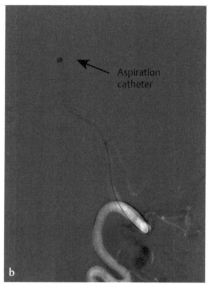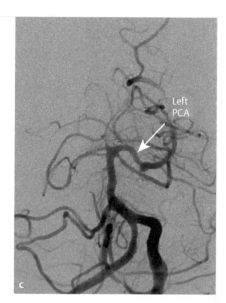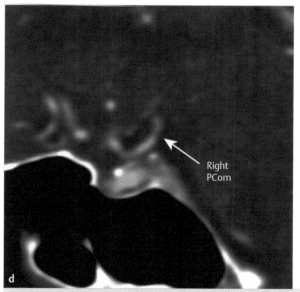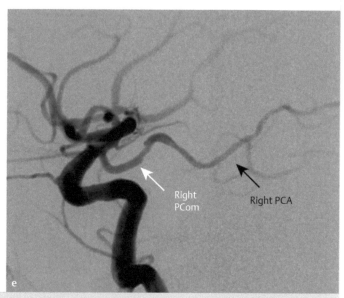

Fig. 15.6 Example of fetal posterior cerebral artery (PCA) variant encountered during basilar artery (BA) thrombectomy. **(a)** Roadmap, left vertebral artery (VA) injection, anteroposterior (AP) view, showing distal BA occlusion. **(b)** Roadmap, lateral view, demonstrating aspiration thrombectomy. The *arrow* points to the location of the aspiration catheter (6F Sofia [MicroVention]). **(c)** Digital subtraction angiography (DSA), left VA, AP view, post-thrombectomy. Patency of the left PCA is achieved (*arrow*). The right PCA is not visualized. **(d)** Computed tomographic angiography (CTA), lateral view, showing a prominent right posterior communicating (PCom) segment (*arrow*). **(e)** DSA, right internal carotid artery (ICA) injection, confirmed robust opacification of the right PCA indicating that the patient had a fetal PCA variant on the right side (*black arrow*), rather than a residual right PCA occlusion. Right PCom (*white arrow*).

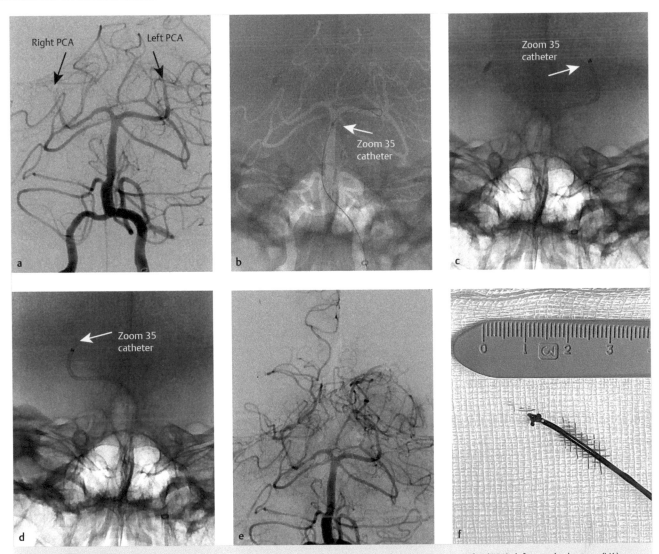

Fig. 15.7 Distal posterior cerebral artery (PCA) aspiration thrombectomy. **(a)** Digital subtraction angiography (DSA), left vertebral artery (VA), anteroposterior (AP) view, showing bilateral distal PCA occlusions (*arrows*) in a patient with the acute onset of blindness and confusion. Aspiration thrombectomy is pursued. **(b)** Roadmap, left VA injection, showing navigation of a 0.035-inch distal access catheter (*arrow*; Zoom 35 [Imperative Care]) into the left PCA over a 0.014-inch guidewire. **(c)** Fluoroscopy showing the Zoom catheter in the left distal PCA (*arrow*). The guidewire has been removed. Aspiration thrombectomy is performed. **(d)** Fluoroscopy showing the Zoom catheter now in the right distal PCA (*arrow*). **(e)** DSA, left VA injection, post-thrombectomy, showing a fully patent right PCA. The left PCA has a more distal P4 occlusion; this location is too distal for further thrombectomy attempts. **(f)** Photograph of a clot corked inside the Zoom 35 catheter.

15.4 Cases with Videos and Images

15.4.1 Case 15.1 Long Sheath, Intermediate Catheter, and Stent Retriever for BA Occlusion

A patient with acute onset of disconjugate gaze, dysarthria, and bilateral weakness was diagnosed with basilar artery (BA) occlusion (▶ **Video 15.1**; ▶ Fig. 15.8, ▶ Fig. 15.9, ▶ Fig. 15.10, ▶ Fig. 15.11, ▶ Fig. 15.12).

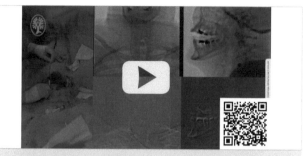

Video 15.1 Long Sheath, Intermediate Catheter, and Stent Retriever for BA Occlusion.

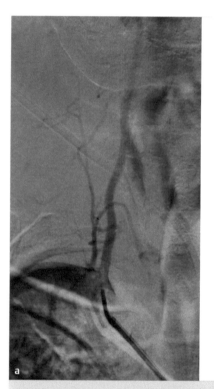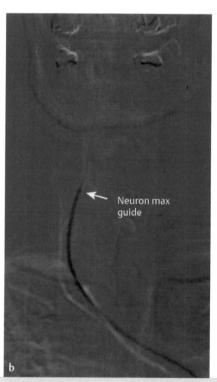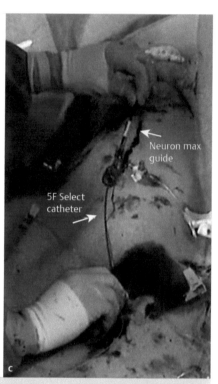

Fig. 15.8 Baseline cervical digital subtraction angiography (DSA). **(a)** DSA, right subclavian artery (SA) injection, anteroposterior (AP) view, showing patent right vertebral artery (VA) origin. The VA takeoff is suitable for radial or femoral artery access. The latter was chosen in this case. **(b)** Roadmap, right SA, demonstrating access to the right VA with a 0.088-inch guide catheter (*arrow*; Neuron Max [Penumbra]). **(c)** Procedural photograph. The *yellow arrow* points to the Neuron Max guide catheter. The *white arrow* is showing a 5F Neuron Select catheter (Penumbra) used for guide catheter delivery.

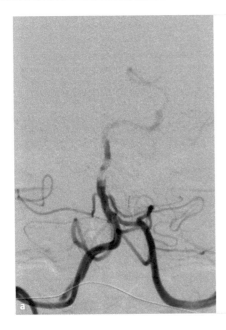
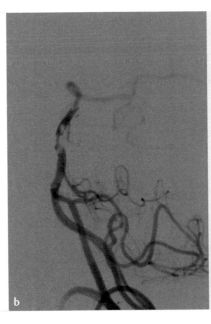

Fig. 15.9 Baseline intracranial digital subtraction angiography (DSA). (a) DSA, right subclavian artery (SA) injection, anteroposterior (AP) view, and (b) lateral view, confirming basilar artery (BA) occlusion.

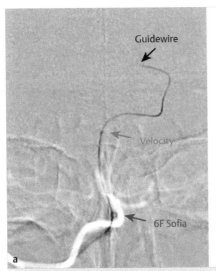
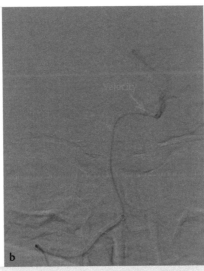
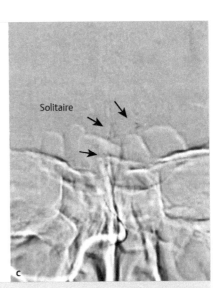

Fig. 15.10 Stent-retriever (SR) and aspiration thrombectomy. (a) Roadmap, right vertebral artery (VA) injection. A 0.014-inch guidewire (*black arrow*; Synchro [Stryker]) is in the distal left posterior cerebral artery (PCA). The *blue arrow* points to the tip of the 0.025-inch microcatheter (Velocity [Penumbra]). The aspiration catheter (*green arrow*; 6F Sofia [MicroVention]) is at the right vertebrobasilar junction. (b) Digital subtraction angiography (DSA), superselective injection, left MCA, confirming good positioning of the microcatheter (*arrow*) prior to SR delivery. (c) Right VA injection, roadmap, showing deployed Solitaire SR (Medtronic). The *arrows* correspond to radiopaque markers on the device.

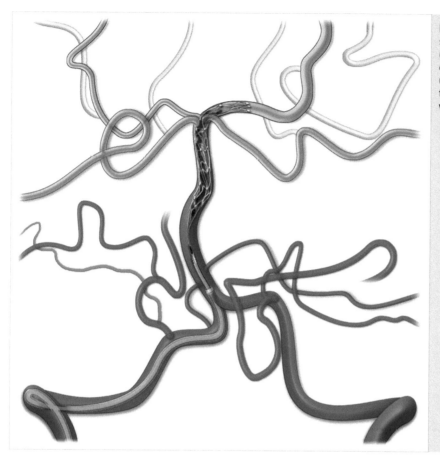

Fig. 15.11 Artist's illustration of deployment of a stent-retriever (SR) device. The Solitaire SR (Medtronic) is covering the clot. The aspiration catheter that is seen in the right vertebral artery (VA) (labeled in *green*) will be advanced toward the proximal edge of the clot while the SR is withdrawn. (© Thieme/Jennifer Pryll)

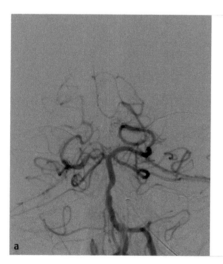
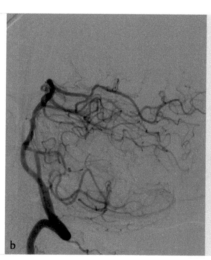

Fig. 15.12 Digital subtraction angiography (DSA) after thrombectomy. **(a)** DSA, anteroposterior (AP), and **(b)** lateral views, showing excellent revascularization of the basilar artery (BA) and both posterior cerebral arteries (PCAs).

15.4.2 Case 15.2 Multiple Attempts of Direct Aspiration for BA Occlusion

This case illustrates a thrombectomy with a massive clot burden, prompting the operator to conduct multiple attempts before successful recanalization is achieved (▶ **Video 15.2**; ▶ Fig. 15.13, ▶ Fig. 15.14, ▶ Fig. 15.15, ▶ Fig. 15.16).

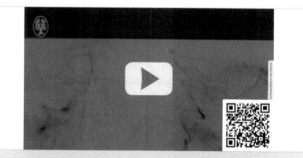

Video 15.2 Multiple Attempts of Direct Aspiration for BA Occlusion.

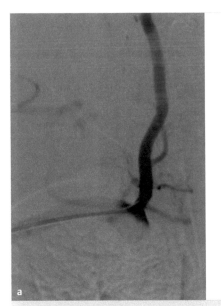 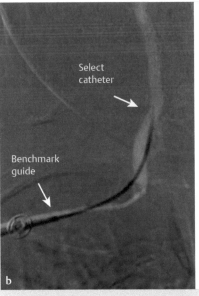 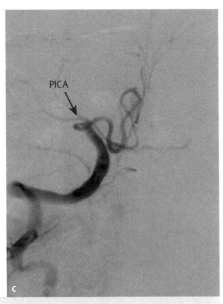

Fig. 15.13 Baseline digital subtraction angiography (DSA). **(a)** DSA, right vertebral artery (VA) injection, anteroposterior (AP) view, showing a dominant right VA. Radial access is chosen for this case. **(b)** Roadmap, right VA injection, showing access to the right VA with a 0.071-inch Benchmark guide catheter (*white arrow*; Penumbra) over a 5F Select catheter (*yellow arrow*; Penumbra). **(c)** DSA, right VA injection, AP view, showing no contrast opacification beyond the origin of the right posterior inferior cerebellar artery (PICA; *arrow*). The right VA distal to the PICA and the basilar artery (BA) is filled with a clot.

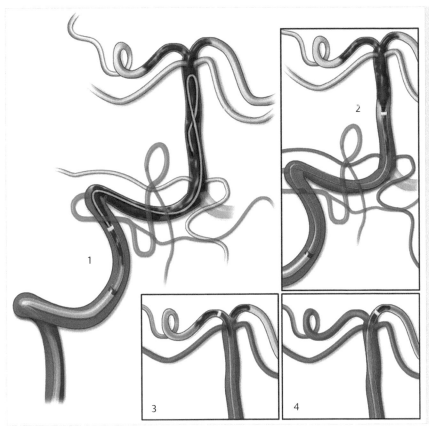

Fig. 15.14 Artist's illustration of multiple aspiration attempts. In step 1, the entire basilar artery (BA) and proximal bilateral posterior cerebral arteries (PCAs) are filled with a clot. The guidewire is seen traversing the clot to provide access for a 5F Sofia aspiration catheter (labeled in *green*; MicroVention). In step 2, the proximal portion of the clot is being sucked into the aspiration catheter by active aspiration. In steps 3 and 4, residual distal portions of the clot are aspirated by placing the catheter into the corresponding PCA P1 segments. (© Thieme/Jennifer Pryll)

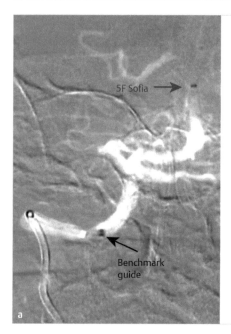
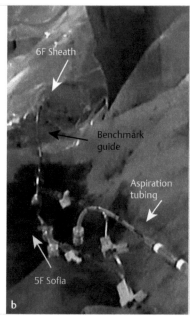

Fig. 15.15 Aspiration thrombectomy is performed. **(a)** Roadmap, right vertebral artery (VA) injection, working projection, showing the 5F Sofia aspiration catheter (*green arrow*; MicroVention) and the Benchmark guide catheter (*black arrow*; Penumbra). **(b)** Procedural photograph. A 6F sheath (*white arrow*), Benchmark guide catheter (*black arrow*), and 5F Sofia aspiration catheter (*green arrow*) connected to aspiration tubing (*yellow arrow*) are shown.

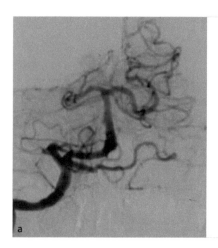
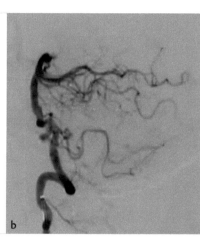

Fig. 15.16 Digital subtraction angiography (DSA) after thrombectomy. **(a)** DSA, anteroposterior (AP), and **(b)** lateral views, showing final recanalization achieved. Thrombolysis in cerebral infarction (TICI) grade 2b reperfusion is achieved as there is persistent distal occlusion of the right posterior cerebral artery (PCA). The basilar artery (BA) and left PCA are fully patent.

16 Basilar Artery Occlusion—Angioplasty and Stenting

General Description

Underlying atherosclerosis is frequently encountered in the middle portion of the basilar artery (BA), at the vertebrobasilar (VB) junction, or within the V4 segment of the vertebral artery (VA) during posterior circulation acute stroke interventions. Primary angioplasty and stenting of lesions at these locations or in combination with aspiration or stent-retriever (SR) thrombectomy following debulking of the occlusion and removal of the adjacent clot is frequently performed.

Keywords: Angioplasty, atherosclerosis, basilar artery, balloon-mounted stent

16.1 Anatomical and Imaging Aspects

- We favor computed tomography angiography (CTA) over magnetic resonance angiography (MRA) because of its ability to depict underlying calcifications, helping the neurointerventionist to establish the diagnosis of underlying atherosclerosis and prepare for potential angioplasty/stenting (▶ Fig. 16.1).
- Perfusion imaging is rarely helpful in the diagnosis of such lesions. However, at times when the CTA or MRA is of limited value, a perfusion deficit localizing to the posterior fossa may aid in establishing the correct diagnosis of acute BA occlusion (▶ Fig. 16.2).

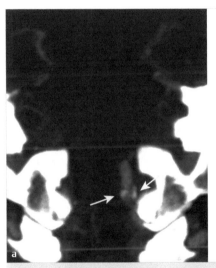 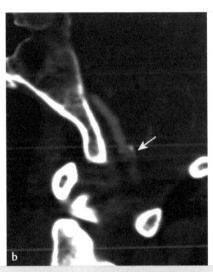 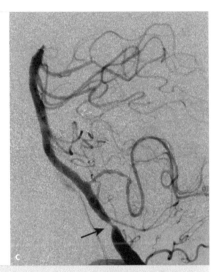

Fig. 16.1 Flow-limiting stenosis of the left vertebrobasilar (VB) junction. Computed tomography angiography (CTA), **(a)** coronal view, and **(b)** sagittal view, showing flow-limiting stenosis of the left VB junction. The left vertebral artery (VA) is dominant in this case. The *arrows* point to areas of calcifications within the plaque. This alerted the operator about the high likelihood of a need for angioplasty/stenting as a part of the stroke intervention and the administration of dual antiplatelet therapy preintervention. **(c)** Digital subtraction angiogram (DSA), left VA injection, confirming severe left VA junction stenosis (*arrow*). Primary stenting was performed (not shown).

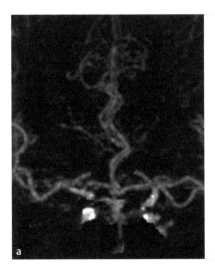 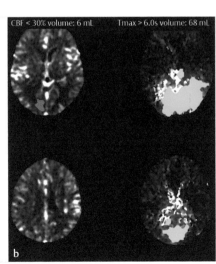

Fig. 16.2 Flow-limiting basilar artery (BA) stenosis with a corresponding posterior fossa perfusion deficit. **(a)** Computed tomography angiography (CTA), three-dimensional (3D) reconstruction. The BA appears patent. It is unclear whether large vessel occlusion is present in this patient who has clinical symptoms of posterior fossa ischemia. **(b)** Computed tomography perfusion (CTP), RAPID map (IschemaView), showing a large posterior fossa perfusion deficit (increased Tmax > 6 seconds [*green* in the right half of the images]).

16.2 Techniques and Key Steps

- The main principles of balloon angioplasty and intracranial stenting are discussed in Chapter 11 (Proximal Middle Cerebral Artery Occlusion—Angioplasty and Stenting) and also apply to posterior circulation strokes.

- Angioplasty and/or stenting can be performed after mechanical thrombectomy. With aspiration or an SR, the clot is removed first, and then the underlying atherosclerotic lesion is treated (▶ Fig. 16.3).

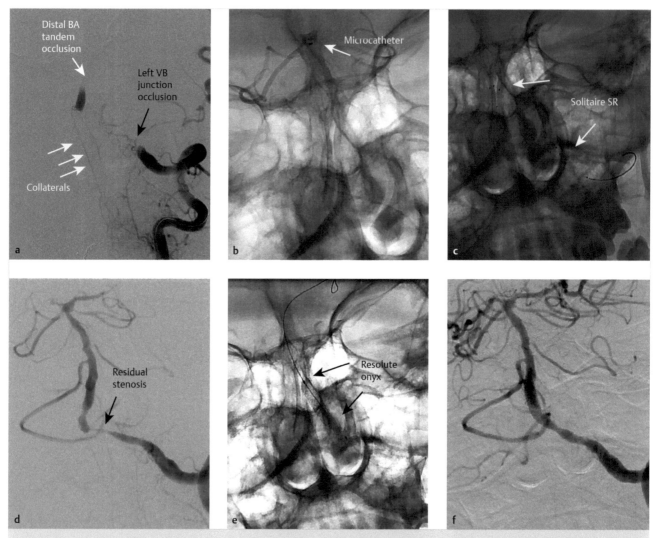

Fig. 16.3 Stent-retriever (SR) thrombectomy of basilar artery (BA) occlusion followed by primary stenting. **(a)** Digital subtraction angiogram (DSA), left vertebral artery (VA), anteroposterior (AP) view, showing occlusion of the dominant left VA at the left vertebrobasilar (VB) junction (*black arrow*). Note distal reconstitution of a portion of the BA via a network of collaterals (*yellow arrows*). There is a tandem distal BA occlusion (*white arrow*). **(b)** Superselective microcatheter injection of the BA. The *arrow* points to the tip of the microcatheter (Velocity [Penumbra]). **(c)** Fluoroscopy showing the deployed SR (*arrows*; 6-mm × 40-mm Solitaire SR (*arrows*; Medtronic). **(d)** DSA, post-thrombectomy, left VA injection, showing severe residual left VB junction stenosis (*arrow*). The BA thrombus has been successfully captured and removed by the SR. **(e)** Fluoroscopy, AP view, showing deployed 4 × 26 mm Resolute Onyx balloon-mounted stent (*arrows*; Medtronic). **(f)** DSA, final injection, showing fully patent BA and left VA.

16.3 Pearls and Pitfalls

- Persistent trigeminal artery is a normal anatomical variant that should not be mistaken for BA occlusion (▶ Fig. 16.4).
- Differentiating between acute versus chronic BA can be challenging (▶ Fig. 16.5). If the lesion can be safely crossed

with a pressure guidewire, measuring fractional flow reserve (FFR) to assess the functional degree of stenosis or occlusion may help to establish the correct diagnosis. The use of FFR measurement is described in Chapter 11 (Proximal Middle Cerebral Artery—Angioplasty and Stenting).

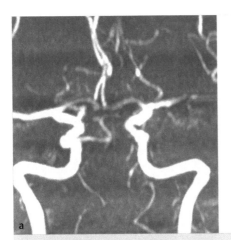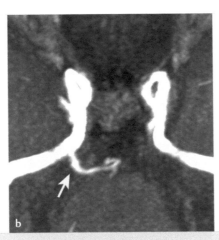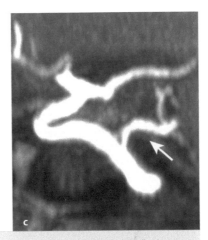

Fig. 16.4 Persistent trigeminal artery. **(a)** Magnetic resonance angiography (MRA), anteroposterior (AP) view, showing poor visualization of the basilar artery (BA). MRA, **(b)** axial, and **(c)** sagittal views, demonstrating the persistent trigeminal artery (*arrow* in each image). It is a noninvoluted embryonic vessel that connects the cavernous internal carotid artery (ICA) with the posterior circulation. The vertebral artery (VA) in such cases often appears severely hypoplastic, and its V4 segment may be absent on noninvasive imaging, resulting in a mistaken interpretation of acute BA occlusion.

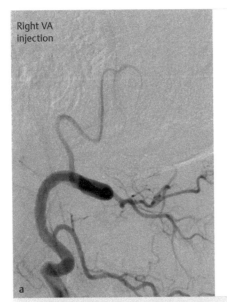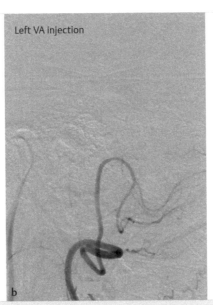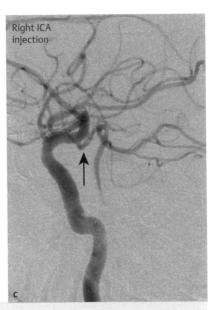

Fig. 16.5 Chronic basilar artery (BA) occlusion. **(a)** Digital subtraction angiogram (DSA), right vertebral artery (VA) injection, lateral view, showing occlusion of the VA distal to the posterior inferior cerebellar artery (PICA) takeoff. **(b)** DSA, left VA injection, lateral view. The left VA is hypoplastic and also ends in the PICA. **(c)** DSA, right internal carotid artery (ICA) injection, lateral view, showing robust retrograde filling of the BA and bilateral posterior cerebral arteries (PCAs) via the posterior communicating (Pcom) segment (*arrow*).

16.4 Cases with Videos and Images

16.4.1 Case 16.1 Angioplasty and Stenting of Flow-Limiting Vertebrobasilar Stenosis

A patient with a fluctuating neurologic deficit is found to have severe left vertebral artery (VA) junction stenosis on noninvasive imaging (▶ **Video 16.1**; ▶ Fig. 16.6, ▶ Fig. 16.7, ▶ Fig. 16.8).

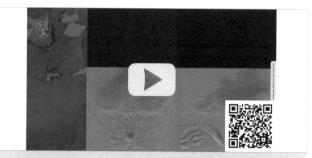

Video 16.1 Angioplasty and Stenting of Flow-Limiting Vertebrobasilar Stenosis.

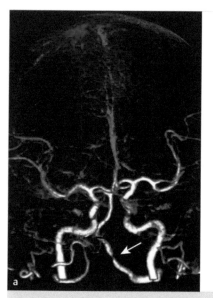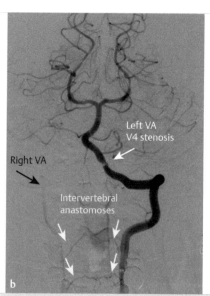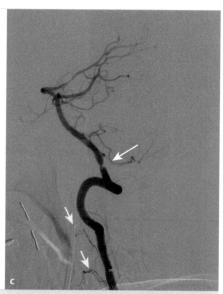

Fig. 16.6 Baseline intracranial imaging. **(a)** Computed tomography angiography (CTA), three-dimensional (3D) reconstruction. The left vertebral artery (VA) is dominant. The *arrow* points to severe flow-limiting stenosis of the left VA V4 segment. **(b)** Digital subtraction angiogram (DSA), left VA injection, anteroposterior (AP), and **(c)** lateral views, showing critical left V4 stenosis (*white arrows*). Note faint filling of the contralateral right VA (*black arrows*) via the intervertebral arterial anastomoses (*yellow arrows*).

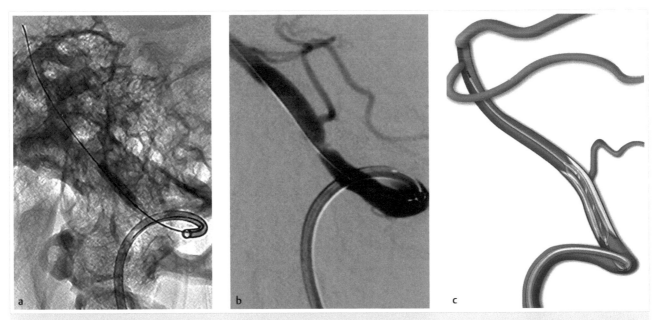

Fig. 16.7 Vertebral artery (VA) balloon angioplasty. (a) Fluoroscopy, lateral view, showing a dual marker 3 mm over-the-wire balloon used for left V4 angioplasty. Note close proximity of an intermediate catheter (5-French [F] Sofia [MicroVention]) to ensure reliable arterial access. The balloon is undersized to the diameter of the parent vessel (4.5-mm maximal parent vessel diameter), to reduce the chance of vessel rupture. Slow balloon inflation (30–60 s/atmosphere) is indicated. (b) Digital subtraction angiogram (DSA), left VA injection, postangioplasty, showing severe residual stenosis. (c) Artist's illustration of balloon angioplasty. (c: © Thieme/Jennifer Pryll)

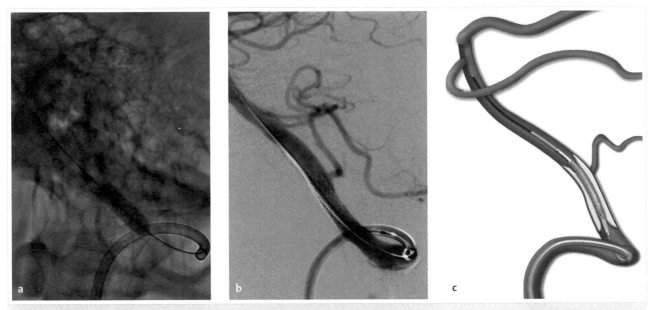

Fig. 16.8 Vertebral artery (VA) stenting. (a) Fluoroscopy, lateral view, showing deployment of a balloon-mounted stent (Resolute Onyx [Medtronic]. Having guide or intermediate catheter access as close as possible to the stenosis is even more critical, because balloon-mounted intracranial stents are rigid constructs and require a significant amount of push force to navigate. (b) Digital subtraction angiogram (DSA), left VA injection, poststenting, showing now patent left VA. (c) Artist's illustration of intracranial stenting. (c: © Thieme/Jennifer Pryll)

16.4.2 Case 16.2 Basilar Artery Submaximal Angioplasty

Severe basilar artery (BA) stenosis versus occlusion was suspected in a patient with acute posterior circulation stroke (▶ Video 16.2; ▶ Fig. 16.9, ▶ Fig. 16.10, ▶ Fig. 16.11).

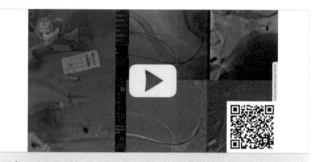

Video 16.2 Basilar Artery Submaximal Angioplasty.

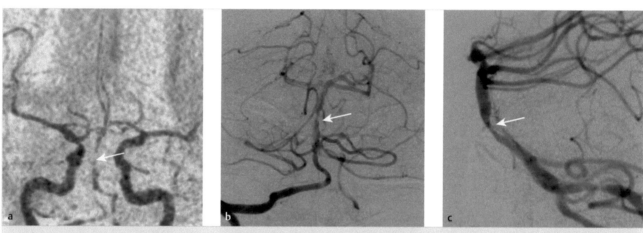

Fig. 16.9 Baseline intracranial imaging. **(a)** Computed tomography angiography (CTA), three-dimensional (3D) reconstruction. Filling defect of the mid-basilar artery (BA) suggestive of flow-limiting stenosis or complete occlusion is seen (*arrow*). Digital subtraction angiogram (DSA), right vertebral artery (VA) injection, **(b)** anteroposterior (AP), and **(c)** lateral views, showing critical mid-BA stenosis (*arrow* in each image).

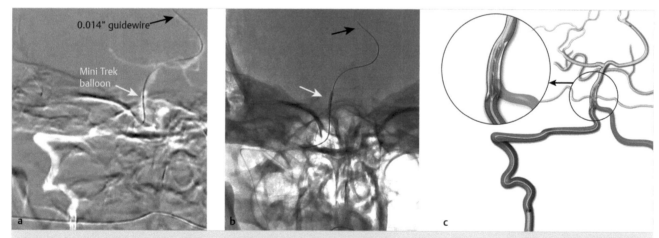

Fig. 16.10 Basilar artery (BA) balloon angioplasty. **(a)** Roadmap, right vertebral artery (VA), and **(b)** fluoroscopy, anteroposterior (AP) view, showing delivery of the angioplasty balloon (*yellow arrow*; Mini Trek [Abbott]) over a 0.014-inch guidewire (*black arrow*; Synchro [Stryker]). Slow gradual angioplasty, approximately 1 atmosphere every 30 to 60 seconds, is performed. **(c)** Artist's illustration of balloon angioplasty. The inset is a higher magnification of the mid-BA segment showing delivery of the angioplasty balloon. (**c:** © Thieme/Jennifer Pryll)

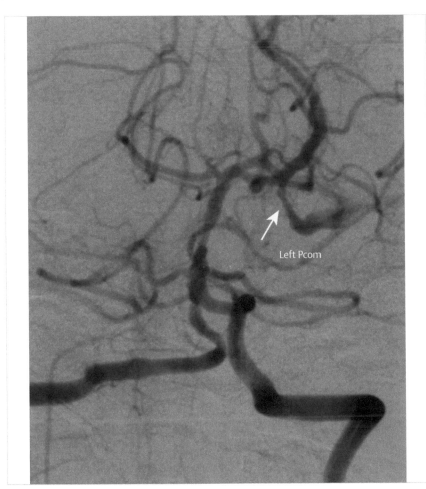

Left Pcom

Fig. 16.11 Digital subtraction angiogram (DSA) after thrombectomy. DSA, anteroposterior (AP) view, right vertebral artery (VA) injection, showing mild residual basilar artery (BA) stenosis postangioplasty. Robust opacification of the posterior cerebral arteries (PCAs) and even the left PCom segment (*arrow*) supplying the internal carotid artery (ICA) can now be seen, indicating that the previously seen flow-limiting stenosis of the BA has been treated.

17 Cerebral Venous Sinus Thrombosis

General Description

Acute cerebral venous sinus thrombosis (CVST) can present with a wide array of neurological symptoms ranging from a headache to deep coma. This rare disease involves acute thrombosis of the major cerebral sinuses. Endovascular treatment can be performed using multiple approaches, including pharmacological thrombolysis, mechanical thrombectomy, and thrombectomy with clot-disrupting devices that are not normally used for arterial neurointerventions. The timing, indications, and angiographic goals for endovascular treatment of CVST can be quite variable, depending on clinical presentation and location of involved sinuses.

Keywords: Cerebral venous sinus thrombosis, computed tomography venography, local thrombolysis, magnetic resonance venography, superior sagittal sinus, thrombectomy, transverse sinus

17.1 Anatomical and Imaging Aspects

- Noncontrast computed tomography (CT) combined with CT venography (CTV) or magnetic resonance imaging (MRI) with magnetic resonance venography (MRV) are the two main imaging modalities that help establish the correct diagnosis of acute CVST (▶ Fig. 17.1 and ▶ Fig. 17.2).
- Intracranial hemorrhage can be present, often observed along the affected dural sinuses and can be unilateral or bilateral (▶ Fig. 17.1). It should be noted that the presence of hemorrhage is not a contraindication for systemic anticoagulation in CVST, which is currently considered first-line medical management.
- Indications and optimal timing of endovascular treatment of CVST are not well defined. Depending on the severity and progression of symptoms and the location of the thrombus, immediate endovascular intervention versus a more conservative approach with systemic anticoagulation may be considered.

17.2 Techniques and Key Steps

- A variety of tools and approaches can be used, often in combination, for the treatment of CVST. None are specifically designed or approved for this rare disease.
- With the advancement of large-bore guide and aspiration catheters capable of accessing distal lesions, we often rely on aspiration as the first-line treatment (▶ Fig. 17.3).

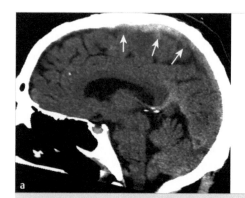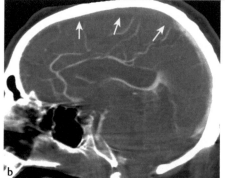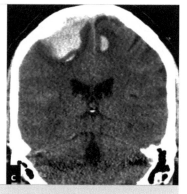

Fig. 17.1 Noncontrast computed tomography (CT) and CT venography (CTV) in cerebral venous sinus thrombosis (CVST). **(a)** Noncontrast CT, sagittal view. Hyperdensity within the superior sagittal sinus (SSS) can be seen (*arrows*). This represents acute CVST. **(b)** Brain CTV, sagittal view, demonstrating a filling defect of the SSS (*arrows*) corresponding to the location of the thrombus in **(a)**. **(c)** Noncontrast CT, axial view, showing a bifrontal intraparenchymal hemorrhage adjacent to the thrombosed SSS.

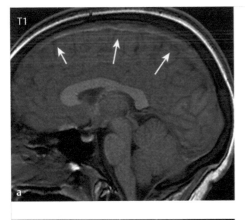
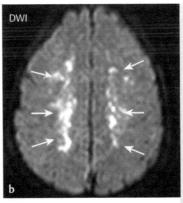
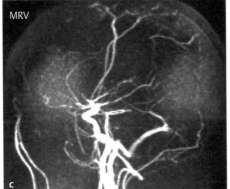
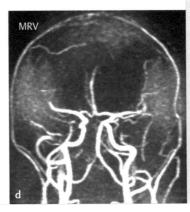

Fig. 17.2 Magnetic resonance imaging (MRI) and magnetic resonance venography (MRV) in cerebral venous sinus thrombosis (CVST). (a) MRI brain, sagittal view, T1 sequence without contrast, showing a thrombus within the superior sagittal sinus (SSS; arrows). (b) MRI brain, axial view, diffusion-weighted imaging (DWI), showing restricted diffusion along the SSS bilaterally (arrows). MRV, three-dimensional (3D) reconstruction, (c) sagittal and (d) coronal views, showing lack of contrast opacification confirming thrombosis of the SSS, left transverse, left sigmoid sinuses, as well as the medial aspect of the right transverse sinus (TS). Minimal opacification of cortical veins is seen.

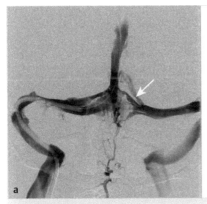
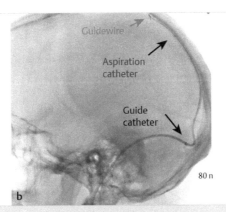
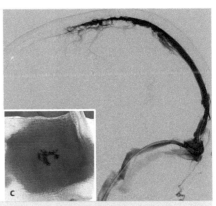

Fig. 17.3 Aspiration in cerebral venous sinus thrombosis (CVST). (a) Digital subtraction angiogram (DSA), right transverse sinus (TS) injection, axial view. A massive clot in the torcula can be seen (arrow). The superior sagittal sinus (SSS) is occluded. (b) Fluoroscopy, lateral view, showing navigation of a 0.070-inch aspiration catheter (green arrow; 6F Sofia [MicroVention]) over a 0.018-inch guidewire (blue arrow; Aristotle 18 [Scientia Vascular]). The guide catheter (black arrow; TracStar [Imperative Care]) is in the right TS. (c) DSA, SSS injection, lateral view. Partial patency of the SSS is achieved with aspiration alone after multiple aspiration attempts. The inset shows clots aspirated from the catheter.

- Aspiration can be combined with a stent retriever (SR) for endovascular treatment, similar to how arterial thrombectomy is performed (▶ Fig. 17.4). Alternatively, an SR can be deployed in the most distal portion of the occluded sinus and its pusher wire used as a rail to advance the aspiration catheter back and forth under continuous aspiration.
- A balloon can be used to macerate and disrupt the clot, which can be subsequently aspirated (▶ Fig. 17.5). We use complaint intracranial balloons, such as Scepter (MicroVention), HyperGlide (Medtronic), or TransForm (Stryker). Some operators use peripheral 3- or 4-French (F) Fogarty balloon

catheters (Edwards Lifesciences) in combination with direct sheath access into the jugular vein.
- Local pharmacological thrombolysis with alteplase (recombinant tissue plasminogen activator [rtPA]) can be used in cases with a large residual thrombus burden despite mechanical thrombectomy (▶ Fig. 17.6). A microcatheter is placed inside the clot and local infusion of the alteplase (1 mg/h) is administered. Repeat angiography at approximately 24 hours helps to evaluate the radiographic response to treatment, guiding whether repositioning of the microcatheter or discontinuation of the infusion is appropriate.

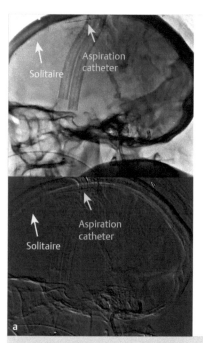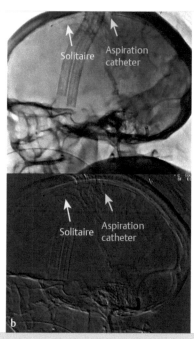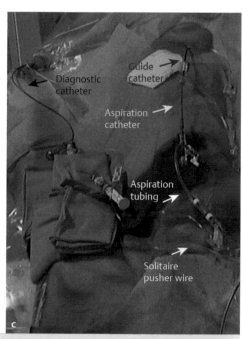

Fig. 17.4 Combined stent-retriever (SR) and aspiration thrombectomy in cerebral venous sinus thrombosis (CVST). **(a)** Fluoroscopy (*top image*) and roadmap (*bottom image*), lateral view, showing a 6-mm × 40-mm Solitaire SR (*yellow arrow*; Medtronic) in the most distal portion of the superior sagittal sinus (SSS). Under continuous aspiration from a 0.070-inch catheter (*green arrow*; 6F Sofia [MicroVention]), thrombectomy is performed. **(b)** Fluoroscopy (*top image*) and roadmap (*bottom image*), lateral view, illustrating repeat thrombectomy passes as the SR (*yellow arrow*) and aspiration catheter (*green arrow*) are placed more proximally. **(c)** Procedural photograph. Venous access with a 0.088-inch guide catheter (*blue arrow*; NeuronMax [Penumbra]), 6F Sofia aspiration catheter (*green arrow*), and the Solitaire's pusher wire (*yellow arrow*) is shown. The aspiration catheter is connected to the aspiration tubing (*white arrow*). Arterial radial access and a diagnostic catheter are labeled with a *black arrow*; the diagnostic catheter is used to monitor radiographic changes in venous drainage.

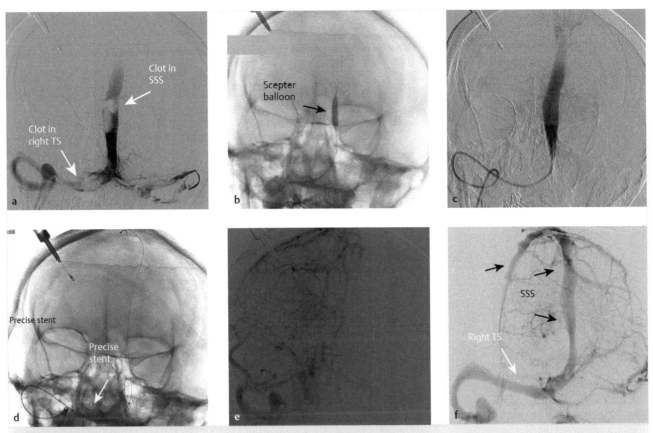

Fig. 17.5 Clot disruption with a balloon and use of a stent in cerebral venous sinus thrombosis (CVST). **(a)** Digital subtraction angiogram (DSA), right transverse sinus (TS) injection, anteroposterior (AP) view, showing clots in the dominant right TS (*yellow arrow*) and the superior sagittal sinus (SSS; *white arrow*). **(b)** Fluoroscopy, AP view, showing a 4-mm Scepter balloon microcatheter (*arrow*; MicroVention) placed into the SSS at the location of the clot. The balloon is advanced back and forth to disrupt the clot, followed by aspiration of clot debris (not shown). **(c)** Repeat DSA, AP view, showing patency of the SSS. The right TS remains occluded. Attempts at aspirating the clot in that location were unsuccessful (not shown). **(d)** Fluoroscopy, AP view. As a last resort, stenting of the right TS is attempted because this dominant sinus was critical for adequate venous return. Deployment of the Precise carotid stent (*arrow*; Cordis) is shown. **(e)** DSA, right internal carotid artery (ICA) injection, AP view. Immediately following the interventions described in **a–d,** poor opacification of the major venous sinuses is seen. Systemic heparinization is continued. **(f)** Repeat DSA after 24 hours, left ICA injection, oblique view. Note dramatic improvement in the patency of the SSS (*black arrows*) and dominant right TS (*yellow arrow*) throughout its entire course. This patient eventually made a dramatic neurologic recovery.

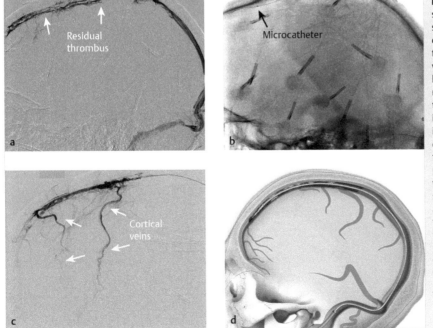

Fig. 17.6 Pharmacological thrombolysis. **(a)** Digital subtraction angiogram (DSA), superior sagittal sinus (SSS) injection, lateral view, showing residual clot (*arrows*) after several attempts of mechanical thrombectomy in a patient with acute cerebral venous sinus thrombosis (CVST). **(b)** Fluoroscopy, lateral view, showing placement of a 0.025-inch microcatheter (*arrow*; Velocity [Penumbra]) into the anterior one-third of the SSS for local alteplase infusion. **(c)** DSA performed the next day, SSS injection, lateral view, demonstrating partial recanalization of the SSS. Note the opacification of the cortical draining veins (*arrows*) that was not present on the initial study **(a)**. The microcatheter was pulled back into the posterior one-half of the sinus, and the alteplase infusion was continued for another 24 hours (not shown). **(d)** Artist's illustration of local pharmacological thrombolysis. The thrombolytic agent (indicated by the *green* particles) is slowly distributed along the channels within the clot (in *brown*). A guide catheter is typically placed in the jugular vein. (**d:** © Thieme/ Jennifer Pryll)

17.3 Pearls and Pitfalls

- Systemic anticoagulation should be continued even after the most successful intervention to prevent early reocclusion. Besides, many smaller draining veins will not be directly affected by the procedure and would require systemic anticoagulation to facilitate local clot lysis.
- Unlike arterial thrombectomy, the optimal radiographic result of CVST intervention is not well defined. In many cases, even partial recanalization (analogous to thrombolysis in cerebral infarction [TICI] 2a) could result in a dramatic improvement of the systemic anticoagulant to penetrate the clot and facilitate its lysis (▶ Fig. 17.5).

- Repeat interventions may be indicated depending on disease progression, which can be monitored with follow-up CTV or MRV. Unlike acute ischemic stroke (AIS) from arterial large vessel occlusion (LVO), which is extremely time-dependent, there is a value of delayed interventions in some cases of CVST.
- Persistent occlusion of the adjacent cortical veins is often seen after patency of previously occluded major sinuses is established. The decision to proceed with endovascular treatment of these smaller veins should be weighed against the risks of treatment-related injury (▶ Fig. 17.7). Although injury to these veins is often self-resolving and of no clinical consequence, they are typically treated with systemic anticoagulation alone.

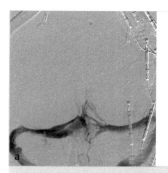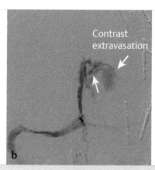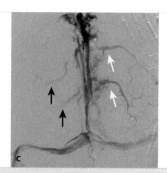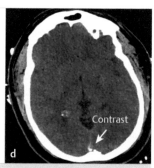

Fig. 17.7 Cortical vein injury. (a) Digital subtraction angiogram (DSA), right transverse sinus (TS) injection, anteroposterior (AP) view, showing thrombosis of the superior sagittal sinus (SSS) in a patient with acute cerebral venous sinus thrombosis (CVST). (b) DSA, SSS injection, AP view, showing contrast extravasation (*white arrow*) caused by inadvertent guidewire catheterization of a cortical vein (*yellow arrow*) while an attempt was made to cross the SSS occlusion. Subsequent injection showed no further contrast extravasation (not shown). (c) DSA, SSS injection, AP view, postintervention. Patency of the SSS was achieved. Patency of the left cortical draining veins can be appreciated (*yellow arrows*), whereas the cortical veins on the right side (*black arrows*) remain occluded. Systemic heparinization with heparin was continued in this case. (d) Noncontrast head computed tomography (CT) obtained postprocedure, axial view, showing minimal amount of contrast staining (*arrow*) in the area of the perforated vein.

17.4 Cases with Videos and Images

17.4.1 Case 17.1 Clot Disruption Using Balloon and Mechanical Thrombectomy

Here, a combination of several approaches for the treatment of acute cerebral venous sinus thrombosis (CVST) is shown. This young patient presented with a progressive decline in the level of consciousness and was diagnosed with a superior sagittal sinus (SSS) thrombosis (▶ Video 17.1; ▶ Fig. 17.8, ▶ Fig. 17.9, ▶ Fig. 17.10, ▶ Fig. 17.11, ▶ Fig. 17.12).

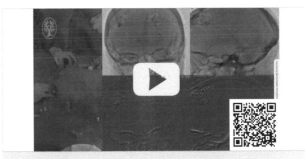

Video 17.1 Clot Disruption Using Balloon and Mechanical Thrombectomy.

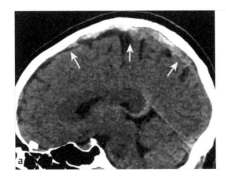
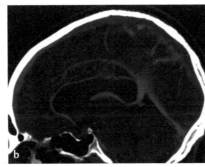

Fig. 17.8 Baseline noninvasive imaging. (a) Noncontrast computed tomography (CT), sagittal view, demonstrating a fresh clot in the superior sagittal sinus (SSS; arrows). (b) CTA, sagittal view, showing a filling defect in the SSS.

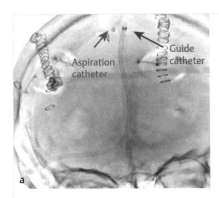
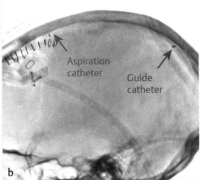
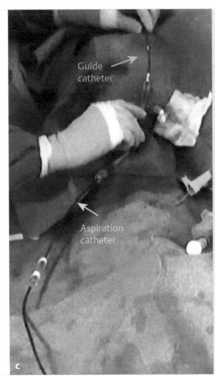

Fig. 17.9 Aspiration of clot in the superior sagittal sinus (SSS). Fluoroscopy: (a) anteroposterior (AP) and (b) lateral views, showing aspiration of the clot in the SSS using a 0.070-inch aspiration catheter (green arrow; 6F Sofia [MicroVention]). Note that a 0.088-inch guide catheter (blue arrow, TracStar [Imperative Care]) is also placed in the affected sinus. Modern highly trackable distal guide catheters provide an advantage of such distal access. (c) Procedural photograph of the 0.088-inch guide catheter (blue arrow; TracStar [Imperative Care]) and 6F Sofia aspiration catheter (green arrow) connected to the aspiration tubing.

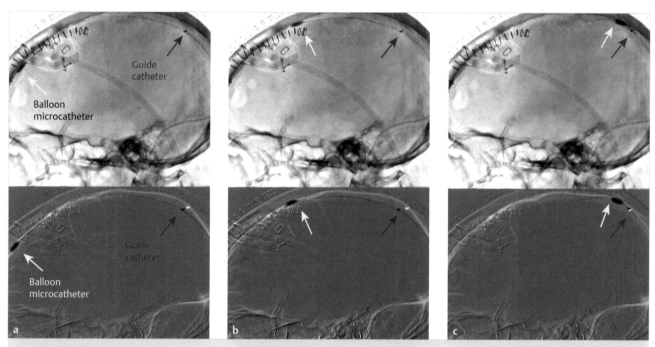

Fig. 17.10 Using a balloon for additional clot disruption during aspiration. **(a–c)** Fluoroscopy (*top images*) and roadmap (*bottom images*), lateral views, sequential images. A compliant balloon (*yellow arrow*) is fully inflated and pulled back, causing clot maceration. At the same time, aspiration is applied to the 0.088-inch guide catheter (*blue arrow*; TracStar [Imperative Care]) that is positioned more proximally in the superior sagittal sinus (SSS).

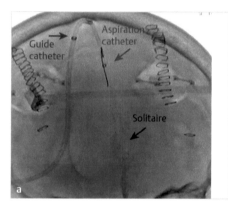 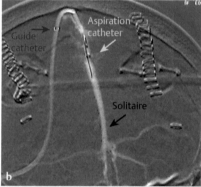

Fig. 17.11 Combining aspiration and stent-retriever (SR) thrombectomy. **(a)** Fluoroscopy and **(b)** roadmap, oblique working views, showing a 6-mm × 40-mm Solitaire SR (*black arrow*; Medtronic) deployed in the anterior portion of the superior sagittal sinus (SSS). Under continuous aspiration through the aspiration catheter (*green arrow*), this construct is pulled back into the guide catheter (*blue arrow*; TracStar [Imperative Care]).

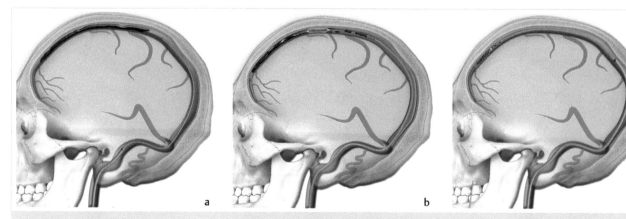

Fig. 17.12 Artist's illustration of methods for cerebral venous sinus thrombosis (CVST) interventions. **(a)** Primary aspiration of clot. **(b)** Combining clot disruption using a balloon with local aspiration. **(c)** Combined stent-retriever (SR) and aspiration thrombectomy. (© Thieme/Jennifer Pryll)

18 Management of Complications

General Description

The endovascular thrombectomy (ET) procedure for acute ischemic stroke (AIS) is the most extreme example of an emergent life-saving procedure. It is often performed under critical, time-sensitive conditions with minimal to no previous medical information available to the operator. From a technical standpoint, catheters and thrombectomy devices are introduced into the vasculature in a "blinded" fashion, without a roadmap beyond the occlusion site. Combined with the burden of stoke damage and concurrent other serious medical conditions, complications are often inevitable and can occur despite all the precautions taken by the treatment team. In this chapter, we discuss the recognition and management of the most frequent and serious complications that occur during and immediately after ET for AIS.

Keywords: Perforation, reperfusion hemorrhage, thrombosis

18.1 Vessel Perforation

- Intraprocedural vessel perforation can occur during various steps of the ET procedure, such as while traversing the occlusion with a guidewire or microcatheter, deploying or withdrawing a stent-retriever (SR) device, or advancing a large-bore aspiration catheter intracranially.
- Early recognition of this complication is critical in its successful mitigation; small perforations can often resolve spontaneously as the occlusion (thrombus) provides the necessary tamponade, allowing the operator to carry on the ET once repeat angiography shows no further contrast extravasation (▶ Fig. 18.1).
- More extensive vessel damage will require immediate additional interventions, such as reversal of anticoagulation (when applicable), temporary use of an intracranial balloon (▶ Fig. 18.2), or even vessel sacrifice as the last resort (▶ Fig. 18.3).
- If a balloon guide catheter (BGC) is used for access, immediate inflation of the balloon may be helpful by rapidly reducing the rate of intracranial arterial flow.

18.2 Dissection

- Iatrogenic dissection can occur when advancing a guide catheter or an aspiration catheter for more distal access or even when withdrawing an SR (in this case, the dissection can occur as a result of SR's pusher wire damaging the vessel). The degree of dissection will dictate whether repair with stent placement is indicated (▶ Fig. 18.4).
- Because dual antiplatelet therapy is typically required for stent placement, the extent of stroke burden (stroke core size) should also be taken into consideration.

18.3 Access-Site Complications

- Given the tendency of modern ET devices to "go bigger" (large aspiration catheters, use of 6 French (F) inner diameter long sheaths or balloon guide catheters), the use of 8F or 9F femoral sheaths has become standard. A diseased femoral artery or concurrent use of systemic thrombolytics and/or antiplatelets places patients undergoing ET at risks for serious access-site complications, which are described in more detail in Chapter 2 "Arterial Access."

18.4 Reperfusion Hemorrhage

- This serious complication is often associated with a large stroke burden (stroke core) that can be seen on baseline (preintervention) imaging (▶ Fig. 18.5). Concurrent use of intravenous thrombolytics or oral or intravenous antiplatelet agents could increase the likelihood of reperfusion hemorrhage (▶ Fig. 18.6).
- A small amount of contrast staining or petechial hemorrhage on postintervention imaging is not uncommon and typically is self-resolving (▶ Fig. 18.7). A type-2 parenchymal hematoma, defined as a large hematoma with significant mass effect, is the type of revascularization-induced intracerebral hemorrhage (ICH) that carries a very poor prognosis (▶ Fig. 18.5).

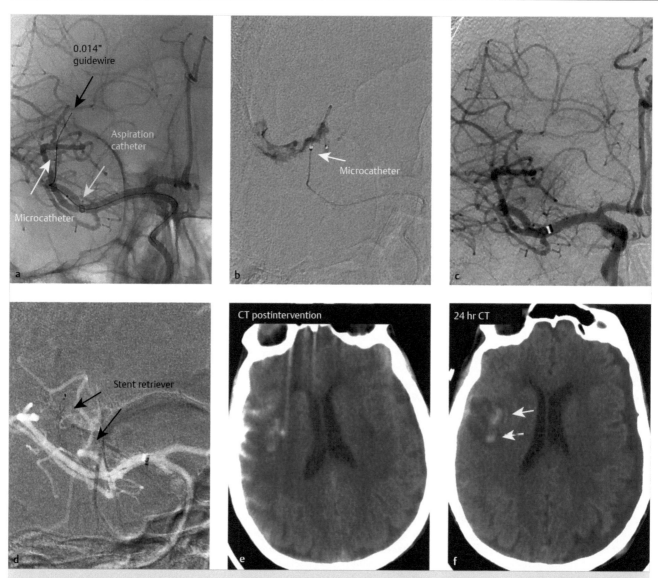

Fig. 18.1 Distal thrombectomy with wire perforation. **(a)** Unsubtracted digital subtraction angiography (DSA), right internal carotid artery (ICA) injection, anteroposterior (AP) view. The operator is attempting to traverse a right middle cerebral artery (MCA) M2 branch occlusion with a 0.014-inch guidewire (*black arrow*) and a microcatheter (*yellow arrow*) to use a stent retriever (SR). The *green arrow* points to an aspiration catheter at the MCA bifurcation. **(b)** Microcatheter injection, AP view, after traversing the occlusion. Contrast extravasation is seen. This illustrates the importance of angiographic confirmation of microcatheter position (*yellow arrow*) before an SR is deployed. Next, the operator removes the microcatheter and performs repeat angiography. **(c)** Repeat DSA, right ICA injection. No further contrast extravasation is seen—the thrombus is providing "natural" hemostasis in this case. After waiting for a few minutes, thrombectomy is reattempted. This time, the microcatheter crosses the occlusion and DSA confirms its safe distal position (not shown). **(d)** Roadmap, AP view, showing a deployed SR (*arrows*). **(e)** Noncontrast head computed tomography (CT) immediately after the intervention, showing contrast material in the subarachnoid space. However, the findings on the patient's examination are improving. **(f)** Repeat noncontrast head CT the following day, demonstrating complete resolution of the previously seen subarachnoid hemorrhage. Small petechial hemorrhage within the stroke core (*arrows*) can be appreciated.

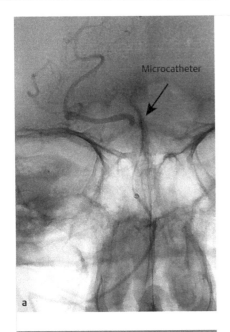

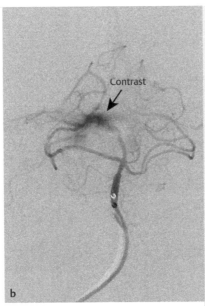

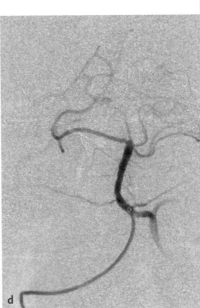

Fig. 18.2 Basilar artery perforation controlled with balloon inflation. **(a)** Unsubtracted digital subtraction angiography (DSA), right posterior cerebral artery (PCA) injection, anteroposterior (AP) view. In this case of suspected top of basilar artery occlusion, with the clot extending into the right PCA, the operator crossed the occlusion with a microcatheter (*arrow*), followed by a stent-retriever (SR) thrombectomy pass (not shown). **(b)** DSA, post-thrombectomy, basilar artery injection, AP view. Active contrast extravasation is seen (*arrow*). **(c)** Fluoroscopy, AP view, showing delivery of a 4-mm × 10-mm Scepter balloon microcatheter (MicroVention) at the right P1–basilar artery junction (*arrow*). The balloon was inflated for several minutes. **(d)** Repeat DSA, AP view, showing no further contrast extravasation. No further thrombectomy attempts were performed in this case. The left PCA does not opacify on this injection because the patient has a "fetal" PCA anatomic variant on the left side.

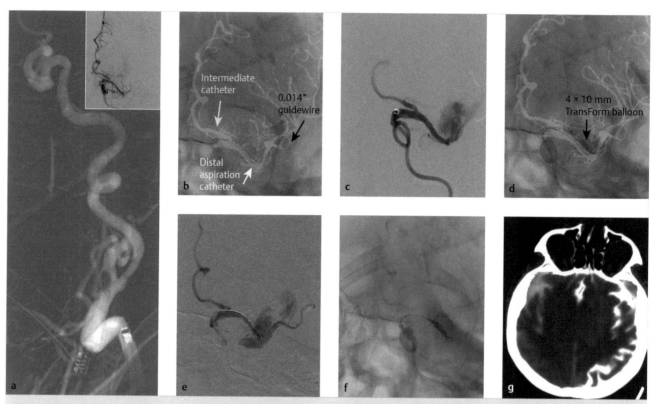

Fig. 18.3 M1 thrombectomy with middle cerebral artery (MCA) perforation requiring vessel sacrifice. **(a)** Roadmap, left common carotid artery injection, lateral view, showing severe tortuosity of the left internal carotid artery (ICA). In such cases, one-to-one feedback when advancing catheters and thrombectomy devices is often compromised, increasing the risk of vessel injury during the endovascular thrombectomy (ET) procedure. Intracranial view, left M1 occlusion, is shown in the inset. Left M1 aspiration was performed, with repeat digital subtraction angiography (DSA) showing a more distal M2 occlusion (not shown). **(b)** Roadmap, left ICA injection, showing delivery of a 6F aspiration intermediate catheter (*green arrow*), 0.014-inch guidewire (*black arrow*), and 0.035-inch distal aspiration catheter (*yellow arrow*) for M2 thrombectomy. The operator encountered resistance during this maneuver. **(c)** DSA, left ICA injection, showing active contrast extravasation at the left M1–2 junction. Focal stenosis with underlying atherosclerosis or a small aneurysm can sometimes be later appreciated in such cases, contributing to vessel injury. **(d)** Roadmap, left ICA injection, anteroposterior (AP) view, showing an inflated balloon microcatheter (*black arrow*; 4-mm × 10-mm TransForm [Stryker]) brought into the left M1 segment to stop the bleeding. **(e)** DSA, left ICA injection. The balloon is now deflated, and repeat angiography demonstrates persistent active contrast extravasation. Additional balloon inflation for several minutes failed to stop the bleeding (not shown). **(f)** Fluoroscopy, AP view, showing left MCA sacrifice with coils. This is the last resort as all other attempts to achieve hemostasis have failed. **(g)** Noncontrast head computed tomography (CT), axial view, showing diffuse subarachnoid hemorrhage with superimposed contrast material.

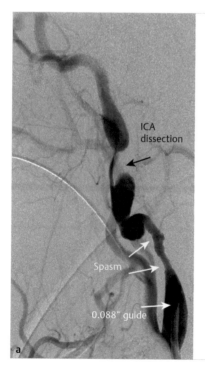

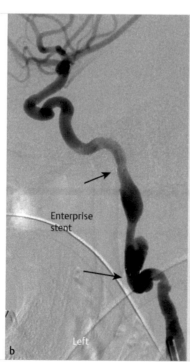

Fig. 18.4 Iatrogenic internal carotid artery (ICA) dissection from guide catheter placement. **(a)** Digital subtraction angiography (DSA), ICA injection, lateral view. Following successful middle cerebral artery (MCA) thrombectomy (not shown), a control angiogram showed severe proximal left ICA vasospasm (*yellow arrows*) as well as a distinct area of flow-limiting dissection (*black arrow*), likely as a result of previous placement of a 0.088-inch guide catheter (*white arrow*) distally into the ICA petrous segment. Given the critical nature of the stenosis caused by the dissection, stenting is indicated to prevent a new stroke. **(b)** DSA, ICA injection, showing patency of the ICA restored by placing a 4-mm × 39-mm Enterprise closed-cell laser-cut stent (Stryker; *black arrows* point to the proximal and distal stent radiopaque markers).

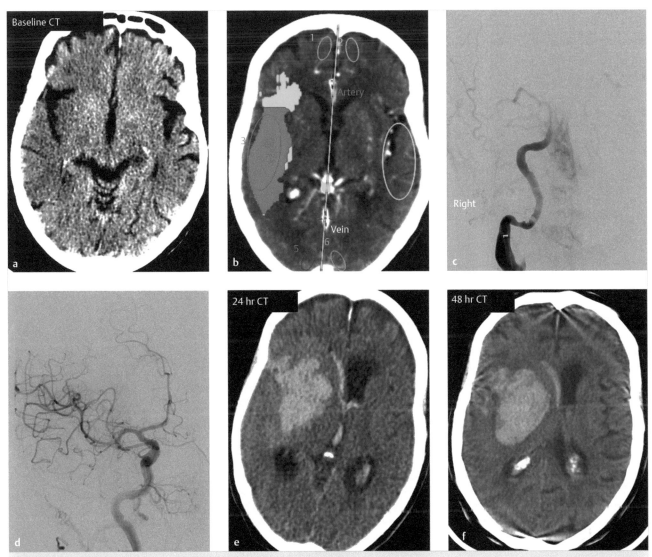

Fig. 18.5 Reperfusion hemorrhage after right internal carotid artery (ICA) thrombectomy. **(a)** Noncontrast head computed tomography (CT), coronal view. Diffuse hypodensity within the right middle cerebral artery (MCA) territory is seen (outlined in *red*). This patient has a poor Alberta Stroke Program Early CT Score (ASPECTS). **(b)** Computed tomography perfusion (CTP) imaging, postprocessing, showing a large ischemic core (*red*) with minimal penumbral tissue (*green*). **(c)** Digital subtraction angiography (DSA), right carotid injection, confirming right ICA occlusion. **(d)** DSA, postthrombectomy, showing successful recanalization. **(e)** Repeat head CT at 24 hours showing a large intracerebral hemorrhage (ICH) in the right basal ganglia with some mass effect. A small intraventricular hemorrhage is noted. **(f)** Follow up head CT at 48 hours, showing further worsening of midline shift with persistent right basal ganglia hematoma despite aggressive medical management. Comfort measures were instituted.

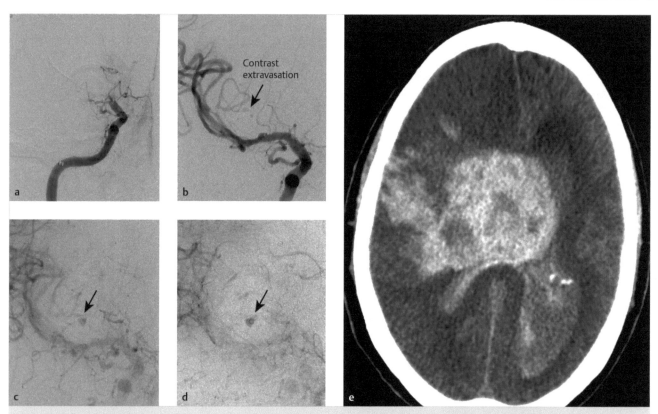

Fig. 18.6 Active bleeding from lenticulostriatal branches after successful recanalization. **(a)** Digital subtraction angiography (DSA), right internal carotid artery (ICA) injection, showing right ICA terminus occlusion. Successful thrombectomy was performed (not shown). **(b–d)** Sequential DSA, anteroposterior (AP) view, post-thrombectomy, showing a small area of contrast extravasation (*arrow* in each image) in the territory of the M1 lenticulostriatal arteries. This angiographic finding resembles the ruptured Charcot-Bouchard aneurysms that develop along middle cerebral artery (MCA) perforators in patients with chronic hypertension. Despite a deceptively small amount of contrast extravasation seen on the images, these areas of active bleeding are very hard to control, often eventually leading to the formation of a large parenchymal intracerebral hemorrhage (ICH). **(e)** Follow-up noncontrast head computed tomography (CT), axial view, showing a massive right hemispheric ICH with midline shift.

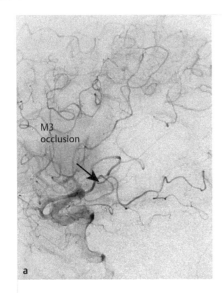

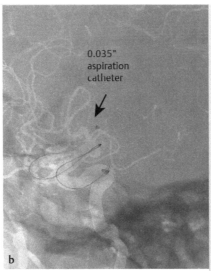

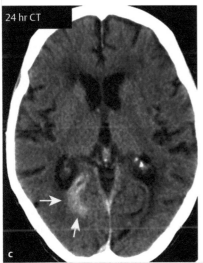

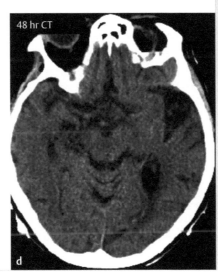

Fig. 18.7 Small, self-resolving petechial hematoma. **(a)** Digital subtraction angiography (DSA), right internal carotid artery (ICA) injection, showing distal middle cerebral artery (MCA) M3 branch occlusion (*arrow*). **(b)** Roadmap showing catheterization of the occluded branch with a 0.035-inch aspiration catheter (*arrow*). **(c)** Head computed tomography (CT) at 24 hours showing a small hyperdensity in the temporo-occipital region on the right (*arrows*). This could represent a mix of contrast material and blood products. Such a petechial hemorrhage is classified as hemorrhagic infarction type 1 (HI-1). No intervention was indicated because the patient had a stable neurologic examination. **(d)** Follow-up CT at 48 hours, showing complete resolution of the previously seen hyperdense region.

18.5 Reocclusion

- In cases when residual clot or underlying atherosclerosis is present after ET, acute reocclusion can occur either immediately during the procedure or in the early postprocedure period (▶ Fig. 18.8).
- Typically, if residual clot or stenosis measures 50% or more of the parent vessel diameter, we consider performing additional thrombectomy passes (for residual clot) or angioplasty with or without stenting (for residual stenosis). Early administration of antiplatelet agents (or anticoagulation in cases of residual clot) is also critically important in such cases.

18.6 In-Stent Thrombosis

- Medical history, including being on antiplatelet or anticoagulant agents before admission, is often not known or can be unreliable when ET is performed.
- Moreover, optimal administration of antiplatelet agents intraprocedurally may not be feasible due to a large stroke burden or other reasons; thus, patients who require emergent intracranial or extracranial stent placement are at increased risk for in-stent thrombosis (▶ Fig. 18.9). Worsening of the neurologic examination findings in a patient who had a stent placed during ET warrants immediate evaluation with imaging, either noninvasive or by catheter angiography.

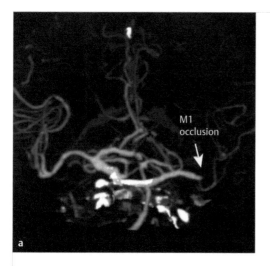
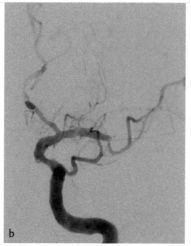
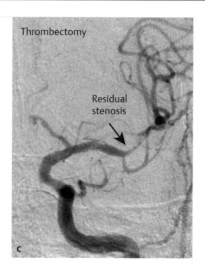
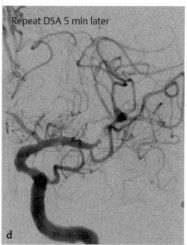
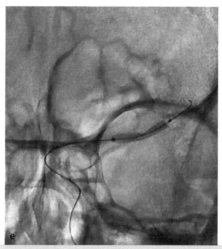
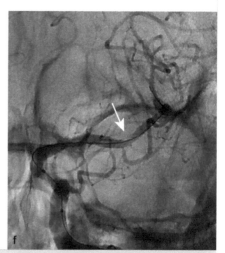

Fig. 18.8 Middle cerebral artery (MCA) reocclusion after thrombectomy. **(a)** Computed tomographic angiography (CTA), three-dimensional (3D) reconstruction, showing acute left MCA M1 occlusion (*arrow*). **(b)** Digital subtraction angiography (DSA), anteroposterior (AP) view, left internal carotid artery (ICA) injection, confirming M1 occlusion. Thrombectomy is performed (not shown). **(c)** DSA, AP view, post-thrombectomy. Robust opacification of the distal MCA branches is now seen, but severe residual stenosis is present (*arrow*). **(d)** DSA, AP view. After waiting 5 minutes, left ICA injection is repeated, this time showing a completely occluded proximal M2 segment. Underlying stenosis is suspected, and the operator decided to proceed with emergent stenting. **(e)** Fluoroscopy, AP view, showing balloon inflation and deployment of a balloon-mounted stent in the left MCA M1–2 segment (Resolute Onyx [Medtronic]). **(f)** DSA, poststenting, showing restored patency of the left MCA. Mild residual stenosis can be appreciated in the midportion of the stent (*arrow*).

18.7 Pearls and Pitfalls

- Complications are sometimes unavoidable. Effective communication among the neurointerventional, critical care, and stroke teams helps with early recognition and effective management of complications.
- Finally, we conclude the text of this chapter with a philosophical statement. ET is one of the most—if not the most—effective emergent neurointerventional procedure

performed in the angiography suite. Furthermore, its value and ability in restoring disability surpasses that of many emergent treatments performed in other interventional disciplines such as cardiology, pulmonology, or critical care. Although many factors, such as age, stroke burden, or stroke severity, are known to reduce the efficacy of ET and potentially increase rates of adverse events and complications, in most cases these should not preclude taking the patient to the angiography suite for AIS treatment.

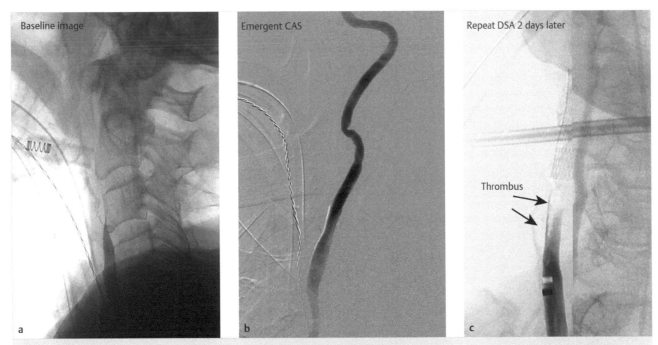

Fig. 18.9 Acute in-stent thrombosis. (a) Unsubtracted angiography, lateral view, showing acute common carotid artery occlusion. (b) Digital subtraction angiography (DSA), lateral view, showing restored patency of the left internal carotid artery (ICA) following emergent stenting with an Xact (Abbott) carotid stent. The tandem intracranial occlusion was successfully treated with thrombectomy (not shown). (c) Repeat DSA, anteroposterior (AP) view. The patient was taken emergently to the angiography suite after a change in the neurologic examination was noticed 2 days later. (Noninvasive imaging was nondiagnostic.) Acute thrombosis of the stent with a fresh clot extending proximal to the stent (arrows) can be seen.

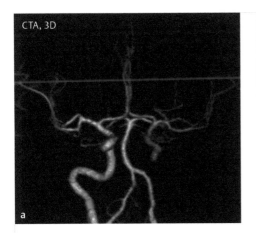
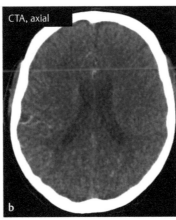
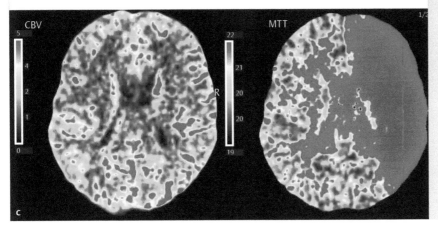

Fig. 18.10 Baseline imaging performed in the emergency department. (a) Computed tomographic angiography (CTA), three-dimensional (3D) reconstruction, intracranial view. The left internal carotid artery (ICA) is not visualized, indicating left ICA occlusion. The left middle cerebral artery (MCA) is supplied via the anterior communicating artery. (b) CTA, axial view, showing reduced contrast in the left hemisphere. No major stroke is seen; this patient has a favorable Alberta Stroke Program Early CT Score (ASPECTS) profile. (c) Computed tomography perfusion (CTP) maps show preserved cerebral blood volume (CBV; left) and increased mean transit time (MTT; right) within the left MCA and anterior cerebral artery territories.

18.8 Cases with Videos and Images

18.8.1 Case 18.1 Acute In-Stent Thrombosis

This case illustrates the management of an acutely thrombosed carotid stent. The patient recently underwent stenting of symptomatic left internal carotid artery (ICA) stenosis and presented to the emergency department with new onset of dysarthria and right hemiparesis (▶ **Video 18.1**; ▶ Fig. 18.10, ▶ Fig. 18.11, ▶ Fig. 18.12, ▶ Fig. 18.13).

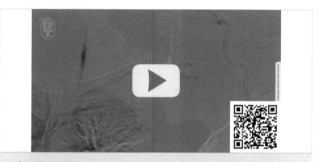

Video 18.1 Acute In-Stent Thrombosis.

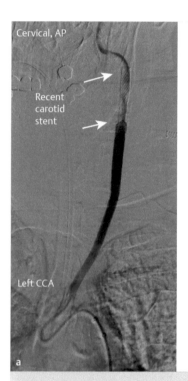
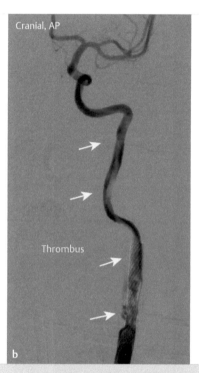
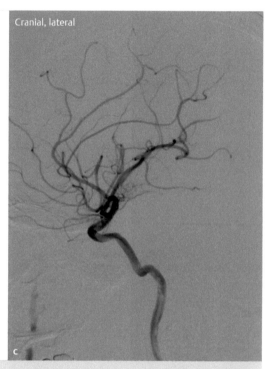

Fig. 18.11 Baseline digital subtraction angiography (DSA). **(a)** DSA, left common carotid artery injection, anteroposterior (AP) view, showing a recently placed stent in the left carotid artery (*white arrows*; Wallstent [Boston Scientific]). A large amount of clot is seen within and distal to the stent. DSA, left common carotid artery injection, **(b)** AP, and **(c)**. lateral views, showing the clot extending to the petrous internal carotid artery (ICA) segment (*yellow arrows* in **b**). The intracranial vasculature is patent.

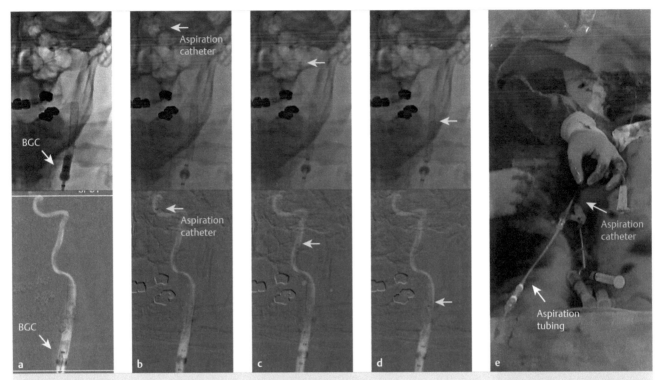

Fig. 18.12 Clot aspiration using a balloon guide catheter (BGC). **(a)** Live fluoroscopy image (*top*) and roadmap image (*bottom*), anteroposterior (AP) view, showing placement of a BGC (*yellow arrow*; Walrus [Q'Apel Medical]) just proximal to the thrombosed stent. The balloon is inflated before aspiration is started. **(b–d)** Sequential images, live fluoroscopy images (*top*) and roadmap images (*bottom*), AP views, demonstrating a 0.070-inch aspiration catheter (*green arrow*; 6F Sofia [MicroVention]) used to aspirate the clot by slowly withdrawing the catheter with continuous aspiration applied. **(e)** Procedural image, showing the aspiration catheter (*green arrow*) connected to aspiration tubing (*white arrow*) for continuous aspiration as the catheter is slowly withdrawn.

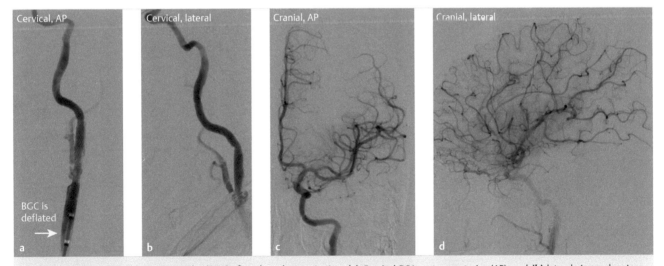

Fig. 18.13 Digital subtraction angiography (DSA) after thrombus aspiration. **(a)** Cervical DSA, anteroposterior (AP), and **(b)** lateral views, showing restored patency of the internal carotid artery (ICA). A minimal residual amount of clot can be seen within the stent. The balloon guide catheter (BGC) is deflated in **a** (*arrow*). Cranial DSA, **(c)** AP, and **(d)** lateral views, confirming no major distal embolization. Using a BGC is critically important in such cases, as clot debris could cause distal embolization without adequate flow arrest. The use of an Mo.Ma proximal cerebral protection device (Medtronic) is not feasible in such cases because access to the external carotid artery is covered by a carotid stent.

18.8.2 Case 18.2 MCA Perforation during Thrombectomy

In this case, we review one of the most serious complications that can occur during endovascular thrombectomy (ET)–vessel perforation. Even with the most rapid and effective response to control the bleeding, outcomes in such a scenario can be poor (▶ **Video 18.2**; ▶ Fig. 18.14, ▶ Fig. 18.15, ▶ Fig. 18.16, ▶ Fig. 18.17, ▶ Fig. 18.18, ▶ Fig. 18.19).

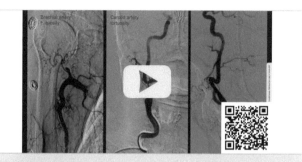

Video 18.2 MCA Perforation during Thrombectomy.

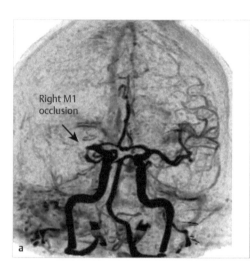
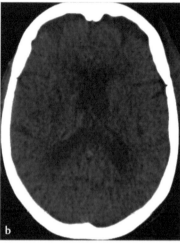

Fig. 18.14 Baseline noninvasive imaging. **(a)** Computed tomographic angiography (CTA), three-dimensional (3D) reconstruction, intracranial view, showing right middle cerebral artery (MCA) M1 occlusion (*arrow*). **(b)** Noncontrast computed tomography (CT), axial view. A favorable Alberta Stroke Program Early CT Score (ASPECTS) profile is seen in this case.

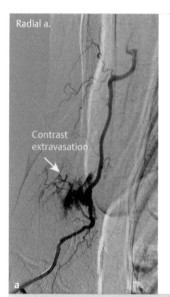
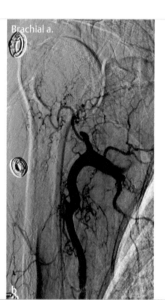
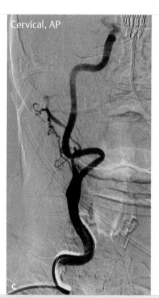
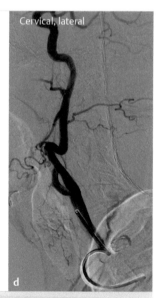

Fig. 18.15 Establishing access. **(a)** Digital subtraction angiography (DSA), right radial artery injection, showing very tortuous and diseased appearance of the radial and brachial arteries. Active contrast extravasation (*arrow*) can be seen as a result of arterial injury, possibly from guide catheter manipulation. This can be effectively controlled with manual pressure (not shown). **(b)** DSA, brachial artery injection, showing severe tortuosity of the brachial artery. Cervical DSA, **(c)** anteroposterior (AP), and **(d)** lateral views, further demonstrating tortuosity of the cervical vasculature. In such cases, the operator often encounters additional resistance and loses accurate tactile feedback during intracranial manipulations.

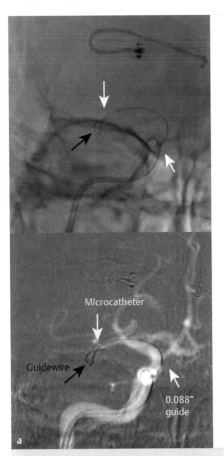
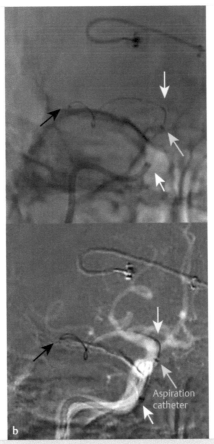
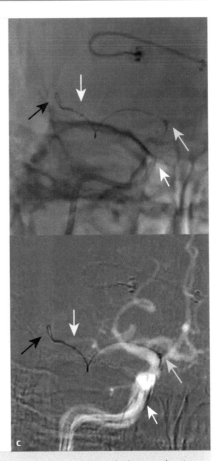

Fig. 18.16 Traversing the right M1 occlusion. **(a–c)** Sequential images, fluoroscopy (*top*) and roadmap (*bottom*) anteroposterior (AP) views, showing a "J"-shaped 0.014-inch guidewire (*black arrow*) and microcatheter (*yellow arrow*) traversing the occlusion. Note how a 0.088-inch guide catheter (*white arrow*) that is initially located in the cavernous internal carotid artery (ICA) segment in **a** is pushed back into the petrous segment in **b,c**, indicating significant resistance encountered by the operator while traversing the lesion. A 0.070-inch aspiration catheter (*green arrow*) is thus advanced farther in **b** and **c** to help overcome the resistance.

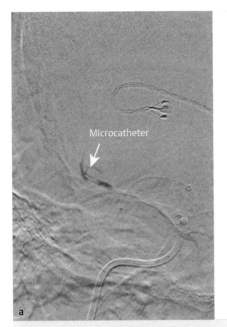
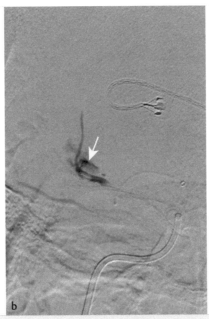
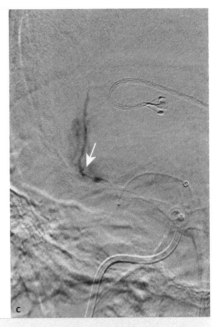

Fig. 18.17 Microcatheter injection. **(a–c)** Digital subtraction angiography (DSA), sequential images, superselective injection through the microcatheter (*arrow*). Active contrast extravasation is seen, indicating proximal M2 middle cerebral artery (MCA) branch perforation.

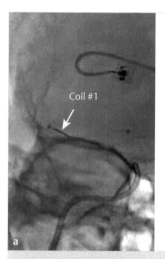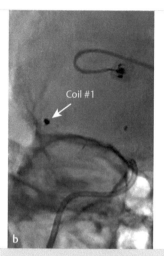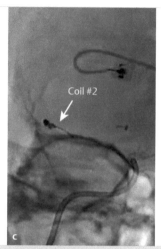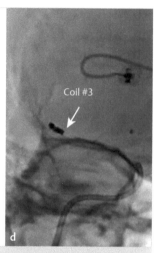

Fig. 18.18 Right middle cerebral artery (MCA) sacrifice with coils. Fluoroscopy, anteroposterior (AP) view, showing **(a)** delivery and **(b)** deployment of a first coil (*arrow* in each image). Depending on the size of the microcatheter used, different coils can be selected so that exchange for a different type of a microcatheter can be avoided. **(c)** Fluoroscopy, AP view, showing delivery of a second coil (*arrow*). **(d)** Fluoroscopy, AP view, showing a third coil (*arrow*) used to close the suspected site of MCA perforation. Only after three coils are successfully deployed, will the operator perform control digital subtraction angiography (DSA) to rapidly stop active bleeding from the rupture point. Faint continuous contrast extravasation is noted, and additional coils are placed (not shown).

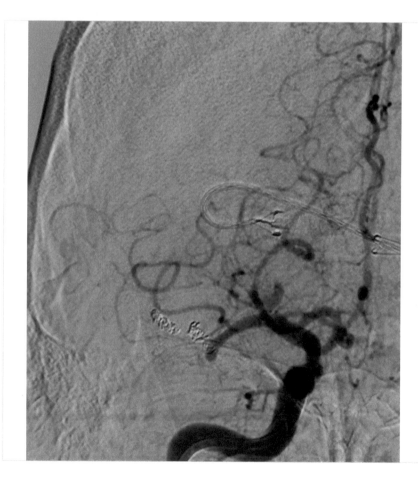

Fig. 18.19 Digital subtraction angiography (DSA) after middle cerebral artery (MCA) sacrifice. DSA, anteroposterior (AP) view, right internal carotid artery (ICA) injection, showing no further contrast extravasation. Unfortunately, with persistent blockage of the right MCA, the outcome in this case will remain poor.

Index

Note: Page numbers set **bold** or *italic* indicate headings or figures, respectively.